OVERCOMING CHRONIC PAIN

2nd Edition

A self-help guide using cognitive behavioural techniques

O
OVERCOMING

FRANCES COLE, HELEN MACDONALD
AND CATHERINE CARUS

ROBINSON

ROBINSON

First published in Great Britain in 2020 by Robinson

Illustrations on pages 55, 69, 116(b), 128, 176, 182, 194, 212, 253, 276, 310, 319, 334 by David Andrassy
Ribbon and magnifying glass images © iStock
All other illustrations by Liane Payne unless otherwise stated

Previous edition *Overcoming Chronic Pain* written by Frances Cole, Helen Macdonald, Catherine Carus and Hazel Howden-Leach published by Robinson, an imprint of Constable & Robinson Ltd, 2005

3 5 7 9 10 8 6 4 2

A CIP catalogue record for this book is available from the British Library.

IMPORTANT NOTE
This book is not intended as a substitute for medical advice or treatment. Any person with a condition requiring medical attention should consult a qualified medical practitioner or suitable therapist.

ISBN: 978-1-47214-263-4

Typeset in Bembo by Initial Typesetting Services, Edinburgh
Printed and bound in Great Britain by Clays Ltd, Elcograf S.p.A.

Papers used by Robinson are from well-managed forests and other responsible sources.

FSC
www.fsc.org
MIX
Paper from responsible sources
FSC® C104740

Robinson
An imprint of
Little, Brown Book Group
Carmelite House
50 Victoria Embankment
London EC4Y 0DZ

An Hachette UK Company
www.hachette.co.uk
www.littlebrown.co.uk

This book is dedicated to all people with chronic pain, their families and carers, and the healthcare professionals who support them to find better lives and better times.

Contents

Foreword ix

People's stories xiii

Introduction: Discovering new paths to live well with chronic pain 1

1. Changing the impact of pain 6
2. Acceptance and moving on 31
3. Knowing more about pain and the brain 52
4. Support for self-management 82
5. Reaching goals and creating rewards 110
6. Balancing daily activities through pacing 125
7. Being fitter and staying active 150
8. Relaxing more easily 174
9. Sleeping well 190
10. Communication and sharing concerns 212
11. Sexual relations and intimacy 231
12. Managing anxiety, worry and fears 237
13. Ways to manage anger, irritability and frustration 267

14. Coping with low mood, depression and loss 290
15. Managing setbacks and planning for the future 319

Resources 349
Appendix 361
Index 383

Foreword

Chronic pain has become one of the leading challenges to health in the world today, both for people who struggle with it and for those who support them. The condition itself does not kill people, yet it causes much misery, grief and harm to the individual, the community and society as a whole. The long-standing and current concern is around unsafe use of prescribed medicines, especially strong opioids and gabapentinoids. There continue to be worrying figures about the number of people who die as a result of using strong opioid medicines. Sadly, in the USA, this has exceeded half a million deaths in the last ten years, and the rate is still climbing, with 49,000 deaths in 2018.

Research is unravelling the knotty problems of why pain persists and why there is no curative treatment as yet. We know more about the problems of chronic pain and its devastating impact on the health of many people. Medical research has focused on medical and physical treatments, with minimal positive outcomes. In the recent decade, research on a balanced approach to person-focused care, including biological, psychological and social factors, is showing more promise of helpful change. The evidence at present shows that this holistic approach leads to a better quality of life, with individuals being more able to cope well with pain.

Self-management enables people with pain or long-term health conditions to focus their efforts on improving their lives. This means finding ways of growing their own physical and emotional health, working towards a more kindly and compassionate sense of self, and re-engaging with social- and work-life roles. Learning about the impact of pain on thoughts, emotions and behaviours, along with one's life situation, means having a more useful understanding of what can be changed. It means having a willingness to learn and experiment with some useful skills, new ideas and resources. It is about developing a readiness to work with oneself, with healthcare professionals as needed, and with other support. Ultimately, it is about a journey of valuable discovery of oneself, health and wellness, and the best of life's possibilities.

This book is a resource that tries to capture the essence of cognitive behavioural therapies; how they are based on current evidence; and how they can help work towards positive valued changes for better health. These approaches include building self-confidence in using kindness- and compassion-focused approaches.

Over two decades, all the authors have started, grown and energised a range of pain management programmes in healthcare settings in the UK, trained numerous healthcare professionals, and remain committed and enthusiastic about working with people who have pain.

Pain is growing everywhere, and resources and investment

in changing its future are falling … so self-management will remain the cornerstone for now and the future.

We hope people with pain will live life well and to its full, with kindness, through exploring and sharing this resource.

Frances Cole, Helen Macdonald,
Catherine Carus, November 2019

People's stories

People's stories we will follow

Here are some stories to show how chronic pain affects people and their lives in different ways. You can follow these people and their progress in learning to cope and become confident with their pain. You will see how they try out new skills to find ways to live well and reduce the impact of pain.

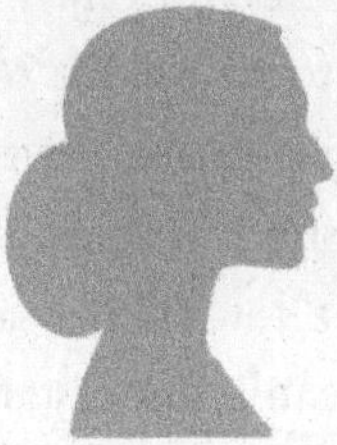

Razia

Razia is twenty-eight years old, with two young sons aged five and seven, called Ali and Yousef. Her husband, Hassan, is a postal worker, so leaves for work early in the morning, often six days a week. This means Razia is left alone to get the children up and take them to the nearby school. Hassan's parents live next door, and often need help as they struggle with walking and shopping. They have arthritis in their knees and back.

Where the pain is

Razia has chronic widespread pain, mainly in the neck, shoulders and lower back. The pains move around her body and some days she has severe headaches. Razia finds that each day is different, as she does not know where the pains will be day to day. 'I can't plan anything,' she says. Her family doctor has told her she has Fibromyalgia Syndrome but she isn't really sure what this really means.

Daily activities

Razia finds that her pain and stiffness change from day to day. Because of this she finds it really tricky to plan her time to get her jobs done and enjoy doing things with the children. Razia tends to rest a lot to save her energy and lessen her pain. She does this so that when Hassan and the children are at home, she can look after them or do things with them. She relies a lot on Hassan and her children to help her out. Hassan can't understand what is wrong and often asks why things aren't done when he gets home.

Sleep problems

Razia has difficulty dropping off to sleep because she can't get comfortable. She sleeps about three hours a night, and most mornings finds: 'I'm as exhausted as when I went to bed last night.' Her tiredness means that she gets cross easily with Ali and Yousef, which upsets her a lot.

Mood changes

Razia's mood was very low after Ali, her second child, was born. She realises that these depressed feelings have come back again. She worries about the pain and what it might mean for her and her family in the future. She feels very frustrated, saying, 'I can't do things I enjoy, like cooking, walking to the park and spending time with my family and friends.'

Treatment for her pain

Razia's family doctor arranged for her to see a physiotherapist, who suggested that she could do some muscle stretches at home every day. The physiotherapist said that the exercises would help improve flexibility in her muscles and make them less stiff. Razia stopped seeing the physiotherapist after two sessions, as she didn't think it was helping her. She said, 'I am just too tired to do stretches in the morning.'

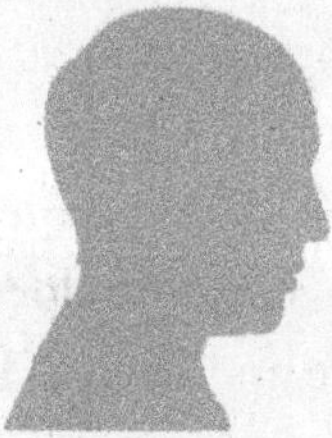

Jim

Jim has had severe pain in his lower back and left shoulder

for over five years. He is sixty-four and has been happily married to Anne for over forty years. He says they are 'a very close couple'. Two years ago, Anne and Jim decided it was a good idea for him to retire as a schoolteacher, but life has been difficult for them since then. Jim's pain has got worse, Anne has struggled with a heart condition. Jim fills his days by doing jobs around the house; he feels this helps Anne out because 'some days she is short of breath and can't even climb the stairs'.

Where the pain is

Jim finds the stinging pain around the bottom of his back and his left shoulder-blade area unbearable at times. His skin feels sensitive and he says that his clothes 'feel tight and very uncomfortable against my skin'. He gets worried when he is in crowds because he thinks that someone will bump into him and make the pain worse.

Daily activities

Now, Jim says that he tries to 'manage everything myself'. He shops every day for food, 'cooks most of the meals', does all the vacuuming, washing and ironing and other housework. 'It helps to keep busy, as it takes my mind off the pain.' He and Anne have a large garden with a greenhouse, which he loves. He now does very little gardening, 'because I have no time and even if I did, I'm too tired'.

Sleep problems

Jim is tired yet has difficulty getting off to sleep, as he goes over things in his mind and worries about what the future holds. Jim has noticed that when he is tired, the pain feels worse; sometimes it feels as though he is trapped in a vicious cycle.

Medication

Jim no longer wants to take his medication. He says, 'It doesn't work and I want to feel in control.' He is worried that if he does take tablets he will 'become addicted'.

Relationships and mood changes

Jim is worried about the future and doesn't want share this with Anne. He is worried that if the pain gets worse, he won't be able to manage everything; then he doesn't know what will happen to them. Their health problems make them more distant in their physical relationship. This upsets Anne as it makes her feel less close to Jim. He is aware that he is struggling to relax or unwind, and is quite 'edgy' at times.

Treatment for his pain

Jim has been to the pain-medicine clinic and tried medications and acupuncture. He is frustrated that the treatments haven't worked and doesn't understand why the pain never 'settles down'. He wants the pain to be 'fixed'. Sometimes he wonders whether he should try physiotherapy, because this might 'help me get back to the things I like doing in the garden'.

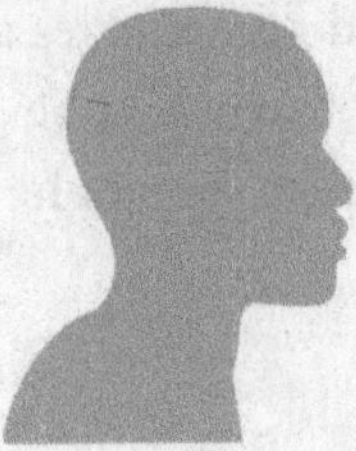

Mo

Mo is twenty-two and living at home with his parents. He was an apprentice electronic engineer and was due to complete his training twelve months ago. While on his motorbike, a car hit him from behind as he was waiting at a pedestrian crossing. He was thrown from his bike onto his neck and shoulder. He felt something in his neck 'crunch and tear' and his knee swelled quite badly. At hospital there was no evidence of any fractures or serious damage. After three weeks he decided he would go back to work, but the pain became much worse again. He had less movement in his neck and shoulders, and his muscles felt very stiff at the end of a day's work. He dealt with this by going to bed when he got home. After two weeks at work, he felt that he couldn't manage at work any more.

Where the pain is

Twelve months later, Mo still has pain in his neck, his left shoulder and his right knee. He sometimes has pins and needles in his right arm, and there are occasions when his left knee suddenly gives way and he can't stand or walk.

Daily activities

Mo finds that lying down eases the pain in his neck but 'it never goes away'. He often locks himself in his room and spends his time 'resting on the bed, watching films on Netflix or using my computer'. Some days, Mo finds it difficult to climb the stairs to the toilet. He tells his parents, 'I am not coming downstairs. I'm staying in my room.' He enjoys takeaways, especially fish and chips, as he says 'this seems to be my only pleasure', although he doesn't like the fact that he has 'put on about thirty pounds' in weight.

Mood changes

Mo feels very frustrated. He goes over in his mind how things used to be and how different they are now, and that he 'lost' his apprenticeship. 'It's not fair that I have this pain. It was that driver's fault.' He is angry about the long wait for the specialist and physiotherapist; also that the MRI scan of his neck showing no evidence of spinal problems in his discs or bones. He has shouted at his friends because 'they don't understand what this is like for me'. To help calm down, Mo sometimes drinks too much beer, but the next day he gets snappier. He often thinks, 'I just want to do the things I used to do; I can't go on living like this.'

Relationships

Mo's mood changes have been affecting his relationship with his parents and friends. When the accident happened, Mo was in the early stages of a relationship with Rob. They had been getting together, but 'the accident ended all that – why would he or anyone else want me like this?' Mo says his friends have 'given up on him' too. Lately, he finds that he has been arguing a lot with his parents about money, as he cannot pay some rent.

Treatment for his pain

Mo has tried at least six or seven different drugs for his pain, but he finds that they only work for the first two or three weeks. He is not keen to try any more.

Sleep problems

Mo's parents have noticed that he stays up very late and then 'sleeps in until the afternoon'. This can mean that he stays in his bedroom almost all day. His mum sometimes hears him shouting out in the night due to nightmares. Mo relates this to 'playing the accident out in my head over and over again until the noise of the screeching brakes wakes me up'.

Legal and financial issues

Mo decided to sue the driver. He saw three different clinical specialists for his legal case. He is very confused about why he still has pain and why his solicitor wants him to see a psychologist about his nightmares and angry moods.

Introduction: Discovering new paths to live well with chronic pain

We hope to share within this book different ways to live well with chronic pain. The book emerged from working with people with chronic pain over two decades, supporting and guiding them in their own re-creation of rich, fruitful lives and so living well with chronic pain.

In this book, we explore ways to support your own journey through change, using this experience of people living with pain and a range of knowledge and skills from health professionals and pain scientists. We hope this book offers ways to turn around the struggles of life with pain and help you become the best version of yourself, even if pain is still part of you.

The key focus of this book, together with its links to supporting resources, is to guide you to live well again, live confidently and find rewarding ways to take action with kindness and compassion towards yourself and others.

We understand, as you do, that living with chronic pain is a daily struggle and is tiring both physically and emotionally. Living with pain is a very personal experience that is difficult to share fully with others, as it is so invisible. The changes, losses and challenges that come with pain and its effect on a person's life often create a fearful, solitary existence. We all share the same problems with this difficult puzzle of chronic pain:

- a lack of adequate explanations for this complicated condition;
- a worldwide scarcity of investment in resources, including clinical and research time, to unpick the many complex entangled causes of it and so reduce its suffering.

Over two decades we learnt from many people with pain about the crucial need to guide them to become confident to self-manage and make better choices towards valued lives, with less distress. This resource is about answering the questions 'What do I do about the pain?' and 'If I am stuck with it and have to live with it, what do I do now, tomorrow, next year . . .?'

The book offers a range of useful knowledge along with practical skills, resources and tools to help you balance daily activities, sleep well, steadily build activity levels and fitness, and achieve key personal goals. It offers ways to come to terms with losses and life changes and accept new routes for the journey in life. It is to discover ways to cope with unhelpful thinking styles, feelings of anger and fear, low mood and manage setbacks more confidently. The book does not offer guidance about medicines and chronic pain. Currently, the use of medicines for managing chronic pain is an area of enormous concern for clinicians and patients. This is due to the harmful health effects of the long-term use of strong opioids and other drugs, information that has emerged and only been understood in the last ten years. Up-to-date information about medicines can be found in the resources suggested at the back of the book.

What you will find within the book

Four personal stories

Jim, Mo and Razia appear throughout this book in the personal story sections, and Maria's story is introduced in the first chapter on changing the impact of pain. Their stories are woven throughout the book to help understand what changes people make in response to the challenges they face and how they rebuild their valued lives. They are based on true-life stories of changes that people have had to make, and include both ups and downs.

Practical aspects of self-management

The practical aspects of self-management are explored in detail, with the focus on the need for a kind and supportive approach to oneself in making changes, so that it becomes a positive journey of change.

The core areas covered are:

1. Knowing more about positive ways to change the impact of pain and discover all we know about chronic pain and why it is so complicated.
2. Discovering the role of acceptance and recognising the grief and loss due to pain.
3. Understanding the role of healthcare professionals' support in self-management and ways to make the best use of their expertise towards your chosen valued change.
4. Rebuilding physical health with activity goals, using enjoyable, balanced (paced) ways to become more physically active and giving oneself rewards for success.
5. Knowing ways to improve sleep and rest better.
6. Using relaxation and mindfulness to create and shape the person you want to be now and in the future.
7. Being aware of the unhelpful role of moods like anger, fear and depression and how to tackle these thinking patterns and take practical action to manage them confidently.
8. Recording positive valued changes with the use of an evidence diary or journal as part of increased awareness of living well with pain.
9. Increasing skills and confidence to communicate about your needs related to pain, life issues and self-management without more conflict or hurt happening.
10. Preparing for setbacks and continuing the journey into a valued future with a positive and curious attitude.

Suggested resources

There are lots of suggested resources online via www.my.livewellwithpain.co.uk and www.overcoming.co.uk.

Greater confidence in knowing how to self-manage means that a kinder, rewarding life with pain is truly possible. It is often a life with little need for medicines and with a more optimistic and happier outlook. It is a tricky path at times. It needs lots of patience to be both supportive to oneself in learning a range of new skills and reducing unhelpful self-criticism. It may mean working through mistakes, staying focused and exploring different tools to help make useful changes.

The outcome of self-management for so many people with pain is rewardingly positive, surprising, exciting and enjoyable, despite chronic pain and what life throws at you. This is why we wrote this book; it is a journey not to be missed . . .

Explore, try, experiment, share, enjoy and reward yourself often; you deserve it. Good luck and good travelling; may you be safe, be happy and live with ease.

1

Changing the impact of pain

This chapter is to help you discover more about chronic pain and why it takes over parts of your life and future. It will help focus on your own needs now and ways to make valued and rewarding changes to live well despite pain. It aims also to help you take control, even if the pain itself is unlikely to change. It will mean taking steps to experiment and use new skills and resources to manage pain in your life with confidence.

How much does your pain control you and your life?

Your pain is real and may have a big impact on your day-to-day activities, your moods, your thinking and how you see the future.

Put a mark **X** on the line below to indicate how much pain is controlling you:

0 1 2 3 4 5 6 7 8 9 10

Not at all — Totally

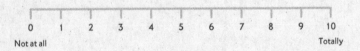

Like many people living with pain, you may feel that it is controlling your life. This book will help you to change this steadily. Over time, as you discover how to manage things differently, you will find that you can let your pain take a back seat. You, rather than chronic pain, will be in charge of your life and your journey.

Getting started

When you have been in pain for a long time, it is sometimes difficult to know where to start and what to do to change the situation. People can often be held back by fears about becoming more disabled or being a burden, doing themselves harm or making the pain worse.

Managing pain involves taking into account what is happening ***now***. Sometimes it is very difficult to face up to the idea that you cannot do everything in the way you used to in the past (→: page 31 for more about this). What helps is to be *willing* to explore and experiment and then use what works well for you.

So how and where to get started. **First, it is helpful to work out how your pain is affecting you now.** This means that you can put effort and energy into changing those areas that really matter to you and **can readily change**. We know this can be tricky, as pain can side-track you frequently. The effort will be worth it in the end.

People with pain who have learnt to manage their pain with confidence, find they have been rewarded with better days and nights and generally better times in their lives.

They became more confident in doing what they really value in their life, despite the pain.

I can now cope with family life much better. I know more about dealing with the pain and I am more in control of it. My confidence has really grown in my new skills, like pacing my day and night activities, using different relaxations and dealing with worries with positive self-talk. I'm now better to live with and my family has a new mother again. I live life pretty much to the full again and in different rewarding ways.

Let's explore the opportunities for change by sharing Maria's story and discover how to understand the impact of pain and see possible areas that could change positively.

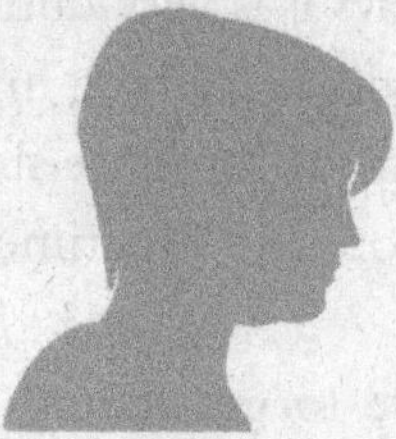

MARIA'S STORY

Maria was a school meals service cook. Now, at forty-seven, she has had a spinal back pain problem for three years since a fall at work. She was married but left her husband twenty years ago when her children were young as the relationship became violent. She lives alone and her four children live nearby. She has seen her GP and several hospital specialists about her pain. She was told that she has a bulging disc, osteoporosis and spondylosis. She doesn't really know what is wrong or what these medical labels mean.

Thinking differently and using a person-centred tool – the Five-Areas tool

Exploring and using this Five-Areas tool helps give you an overview of how your pain controls you and your life now. It will also help you to work out which problems or issues you can change in five areas of yourself and your life, some more easily than you might predict. The five areas are set out below.

FIVE-AREAS TOOL

Body symptoms
(Type of pain or sensation/s in the body)

Moods
(Emotions or feelings)

Thoughts
(Thinking in words or pictures, memories and beliefs or rules)

Behaviours/Actions
(What I do or do not do now)

Life situation
(Past/present, work, relationships, money, hobbies, etc.)

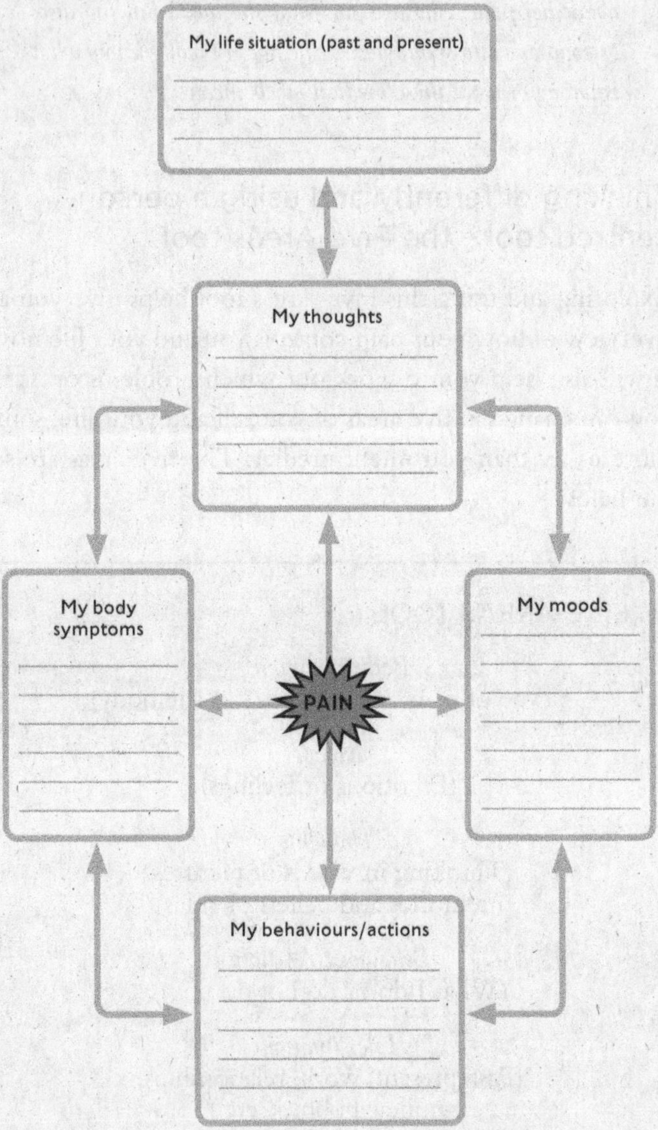
My life situation (past and present)
My thoughts
My body symptoms
PAIN
My moods
My behaviours/actions

Use the blank Five-Areas tool as a guide to work out what difficulties your pain causes you at present and how it affects your life.

> **Step 1**: Fill in each area and this gives you a list of different problems due to the way pain is affecting all five areas.
>
> **Step 2**: Check through your list and then decide which two or three problems you really want/need to change at present.

It turns out that most of the problems due to the way pain controls your life are changeable.

This is really positive news. As you come to understand a problem and learn new skills and tools, you will become more confident about managing your pain and its impact or its control on you. You will find life becomes easier and some pain will reduce.

Let's follow Maria and her use of the Five-Areas tool.

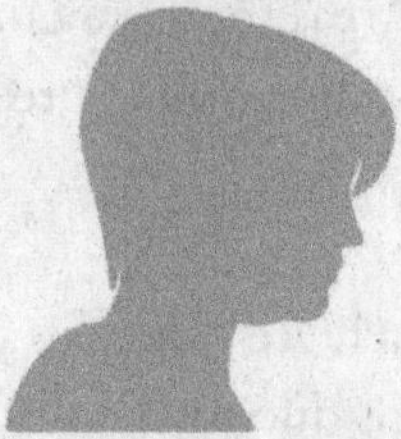

Maria scored herself as 7/10 on pain controlling her life.

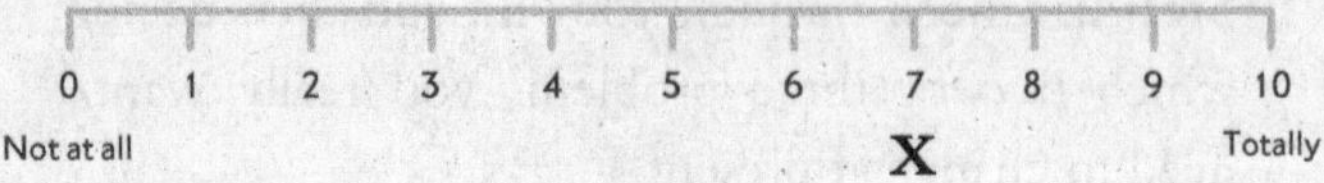

She used the Five-Areas tool to think about how her pain affected different parts of her life and to work out where she could make changes easily.

Maria realises she is no longer the bright, cheerful, amiable person who loves her job and would always help others out. Now she often finds that she can't be bothered to tidy the house, cook meals for herself, or look after the garden. She sometimes gets angry and can be very tearful. She has surprised herself by being aggressive at times towards herself or other people.

Maria's Five-Areas tool looked like this when she filled in each area:

PERSON-CENTRED – MARIA'S FIVE-AREAS TOOL

BODY SYMPTOMS (TYPE OF PAIN OR BODY SENSATION)

The pain 'crucifies me', with spasms.
The tablets make me a zombie.
Constipated.
Sleep problems, wake up each night.
Stiff back – can't get out of bed in the morning.

MOODS (EMOTIONS)

Angry and frustrated.
Depressed and hopeless at times.
So frightened, especially about the future.
I am embarrassed about how I look now.

THOUGHTS (WORDS, PICTURES, MEMORIES, BELIEFS OR RULES)

I am a wimp now, not a strong person.
I would kill myself if I went into a home; it would end the pain.
I hate people doing things for me.
Others see me as moaning and aggressive.

BEHAVIOURS/ACTIONS
(WHAT YOU DO OR DON'T DO)

I spend 70 per cent of the day in a chair or in bed.

I don't cook for myself these days.

I am in tears a lot.

Grumpy, shout at the family.

LIFE SITUATION
(PAST/PRESENT, WORK, RELATIONSHIPS, MONEY, ETC.)

Lost my job and my work friends.

Far less money; always worked seven days a week – I don't now.

Stuck at home, can't get out alone, same four walls every day.

Loved going dancing.

My neighbours now check on me in case I have fallen.

My family don't understand what is happening to me.

I survived as a single parent yet this pain beats me.

The specialist never saw me after the scan test.

Maria's second action was to put an + sign beside all the problems in each area she was keen to change, her priorities. These became her targets to change.

The tool showed Maria all the different ways in which pain was controlling her life. Making some choices about what she was keen to change guided Maria to see what was realistic and possible to change. She knew that after all this time, three years, it was unlikely that her pain could be 'fixed'. She realised that 90 per cent of these problems were changeable, the pain was least changeable, yet this had been her main focus of action.

She realised what she could change was the struggle and feelings of frustration that came with the pain. This could mean she would be less stressed and enjoy more things with her family. She felt upbeat!

Using this Five-Areas tool to identify targets for change

> FIVE-AREAS TOOL
>
> Explore filling in the blank Five-Areas tool to help you see the different issues in how pain affects your different five areas. Then like Maria these can be your own targets to change by choosing the most essential or important to change now. Use Maria's example and what is shared about the tool to guide your activity.

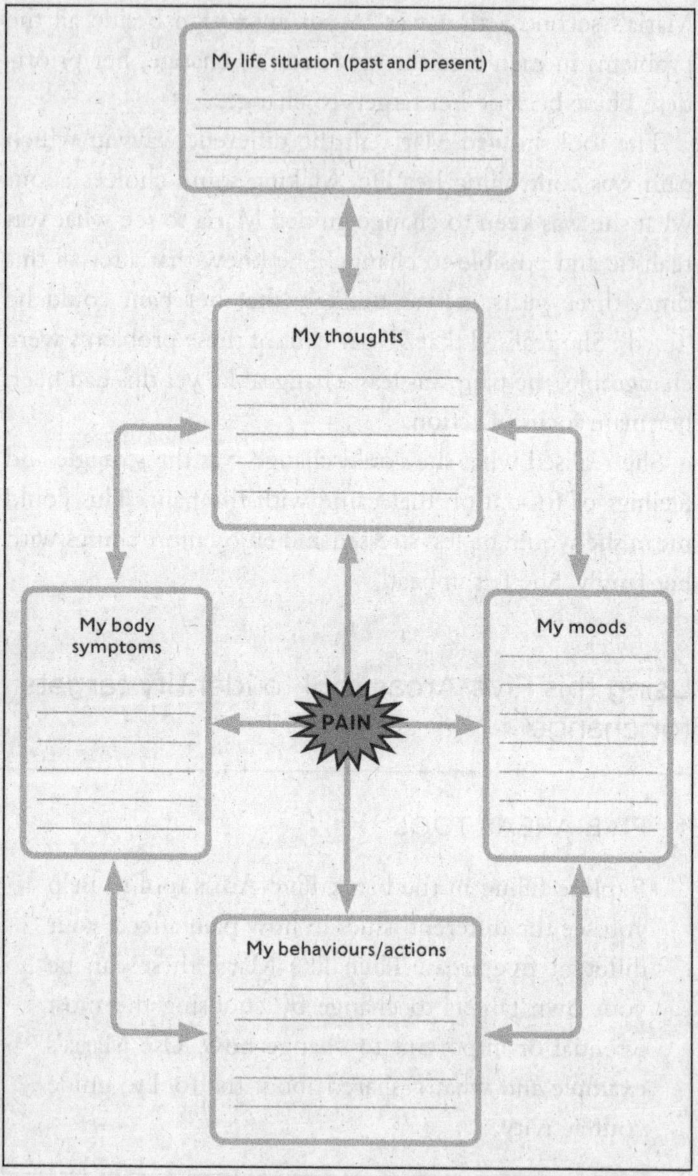
My life situation (past and present)
My thoughts
My body symptoms
PAIN
My moods
My behaviours/actions

- If you are not sure how to get started, look back at how Maria filled in the person-centred Five-Areas tool.
- Use a notebook, mobile phone or computer to keep a record of findings and targets for change.

Maria made a short list from her Five-Areas tool of what for her needed to change. These became her **targets for change.**

Maria's list of targets to change

Take control of the pain in my back.

My stiff back and neck in the mornings.

Difficult to get out of bed/climb the stairs/hang out washing.

Sleep problems – wake with pain/not able to turn over.

Mood changes – feel depressed/angry/anxious thinking.

I will fall and get stuck on that toilet again.

No social life – no dancing/spend all day on my own.

Can't understand why the pains don't go away.

Scan result – what did it say? What does the result mean?

She decided to focus on two problems from her list. She picked these because they were having a big impact on her life. She also discovered that as she started to address these problems, it brought about benefits in other areas of her life.

Explore more about what happened below.

Problem 1	What Maria did differently	Result	Other benefits
Maria had stiffness in her back, which was worst in the mornings, making it very difficult getting out of bed.	She started trying to do a few specific stretch and strength exercises while still in bed to ease her back stiffness.	Maria found it helped make her back more flexible, less stiff, so easier to get out of bed.	Maria saw improvements to her **moods**. She felt less frightened and more confident. Her thoughts became more positive. She started to think that she could manage better and not be so reliant on others.

Problem 2	What Maria did differently	Result	Other benefits
Maria felt depressed because she thought she could not manage at home.	She started to keep a daily chart of the times in the day she did manage fairly well.	Over five days the evidence from this record helped her to feel less concerned. She found that most days she managed well and it was only in the early morning or after a busy part of the day that she struggled with pain.	Maria had fewer worrying thoughts at night, which meant that she could get off to sleep more quickly.

Maria's next steps were to tackle the other targets for change on her list.

A helpful tool to get you started

If you are struggling to work out all the ways that pain is affecting you and your life, then try the self-assessment tool **'What are my Health Needs now?'**. This tool on the next page can help you understand the way pain has impact on the person and their health and the most important needs to change.

Follow these steps to guide your progress:

> **Step 1**: Tick off from the list any difficulties/issues you experience that you want to change now.
>
> **Step 2**: Ask yourself: what are the three main difficulties at present that I would value changing or improving? These, then, are your targets for change.

Sometimes it helps to share your list with someone else you trust. Maria saw her GP, who helped her work through the assessment tool. Other people you could work with are physiotherapists, practice or specialist nurses, occupational therapists, community mental health nurses, pharmacists, family members, friends, work colleagues, local pain support group members and local health fitness centres →: page 82.

If you ticked more than three areas of your life, choose three areas you would value changing now, even if only little changes are possible. Avoid the '*if only wish list*' trap. People often say to themselves: 'All of it!!!' or 'I wish . . .'; this is not possible or realistic. But it *is* possible to make little changes to even the biggest problems – just as it is possible to build a big house, one brick at a time.

What are my Health Needs *now* due to the impact of pain on my health and my life?

- Problems with my walking, moving about and balance.
- My lack of fitness and energy, feeling tired.
- Side-effects or problems with my medicines for pain.
- Unhelpful pacing of my day's activities (a pattern of doing too much, have more pain, then rest and do very little).
- Insufficient pain relief.
- Not understanding why chronic pain happens.
- Disturbed sleep.
- Moods, e.g. depression, guilt, anger, anxiety/worry.
- Relationship issues with partner, family, others, because of pain.
- Sex life problems.

- Not able to work, study or continue working/study.
- Money worries.
- Resolving legal claims.
- Other difficulties that are important to change.

Step 3: Make a note of your three needs or difficulties to help you to draw up an action plan.

Put your three choices in your notebook or mobile phone.

Maria put her choices of difficulties in her mobile phone notes:

1. Lack of fitness and energy.
2. Side-effects from the medicines.
3. Moods; getting angry too often, as I can't do things.

Step 4: Ask yourself, what would you like to be different about the three things you listed.

Maria sent a text message to her daughter Dawn about what she would like to be different or better. The three targets were:

1. Walk more, maybe dance again.
2. Use less medication.
3. Do activities with the grandchildren.

Write down your ideas of changes in your notebook or mobile phone notes:

1. ______________________________
2. ______________________________
3. ______________________________

Stuck? Then try this question to help you: 'What would I suggest to someone close to me if they were in a similar state with pain?'

> **Step 5**: Think about how things could be different if you make the changes to your three targets for change.

Ask yourself, who would you spend more or less time with? Maria's notes made her realise she would spend more time with her family and less time with the doctor.

More time	Less time
e.g. with my grandson	e.g. the doctor

Use the space above to record your own ideas and write down what would be **better** if things were different.

Then ask yourself how your day-to-day life would be different if you made the changes. When you have put down your ideas, you will see there can be a number of reasons for doing things in different ways and experimenting with changes.

Next, think and look for any advantages of things staying the way they are now. This may seem like a strange idea, but sometimes it can help to be honest about the concerns you might have about changing. Don't worry if these things seem small or silly. Make a record of them in your notebook. Here is an example of what Maria wrote:

My positives for change	My negatives for change
Feel good about me	It seems way too much effort to make changes
Doing more things for myself, because I'm fitter	The family will not visit as much
Meet friends and get out	I would have to go out with family to boring, noisy places!!

Step 6: Think about how important it is to you that things change at the moment.

Put a mark X on the line below to indicate how **important** it is to you that you take action to change your three targets.

0 1 2 3 4 5 6 7 8 9 10

Not at all important — Extremely important

Put a mark X on the line below to indicate how **confident** you are about changing your targets.

0 1 2 3 4 5 6 7 8 9 10

Not at all confident — Extremely confident

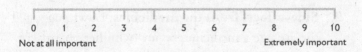

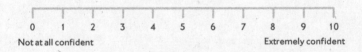

Put a mark X on the line below to indicate how **ready** you are to change **now**.

0 1 2 3 4 5 6 7 8 9 10

Not ready at all to change — Extremely ready to change

Maria's confidence level to change was 6/10 and when she talked with her daughter, Dawn, it rose to 7/10, as Dawn was keen to support her efforts. After thinking and talking about all the good reasons for change, Maria's score for readiness to change was 8/10.

Maria's choices and her first action steps on them:

1. **Lack of fitness and energy**, so she decided to explore the chapter on Being fitter and staying active, →: page 150.
2. **Side-effects from the medicines**; Dawn suggested she arrange a medicines review with her pharmacist.
3. **Moods**; getting angry too often, as I can't do things . . . She thought the chapter on Relaxation more easily →: page 174 would be a good place to start.

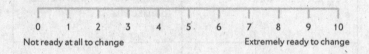

Moving from the pain cycle to the self-care cycle

As you start to make changes to your life, you may find that the pain and self-care cycles help you to be aware of your progress.

On the pain cycle, you will see many of the difficulties that are commonly experienced by people living with pain. These difficulties feed each other so that, over time, they can become worse and worse. You may recognise these difficulties in your life now. If so, you could put a ring around the ones that apply to you.

Changing the Way Pain Manages Me

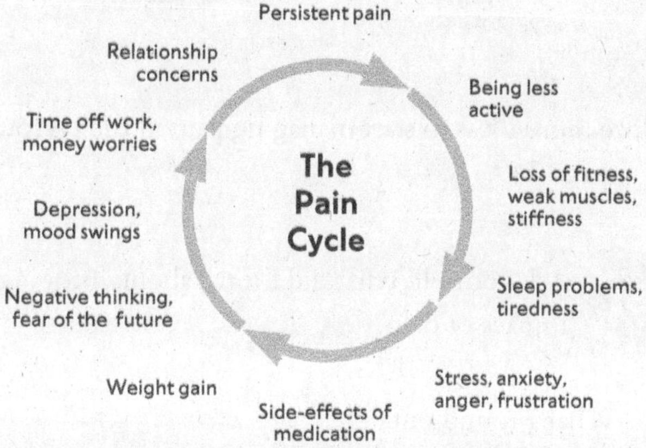

On the self-care cycle there are many of the benefits that come about when people with pain learn to manage their pain with confidence. As you work through this book, and start to make changes in your life, look out for the benefits in the self-care cycle. Put a ring around those that apply to you and share this with other people.

Changing the Impact of Pain

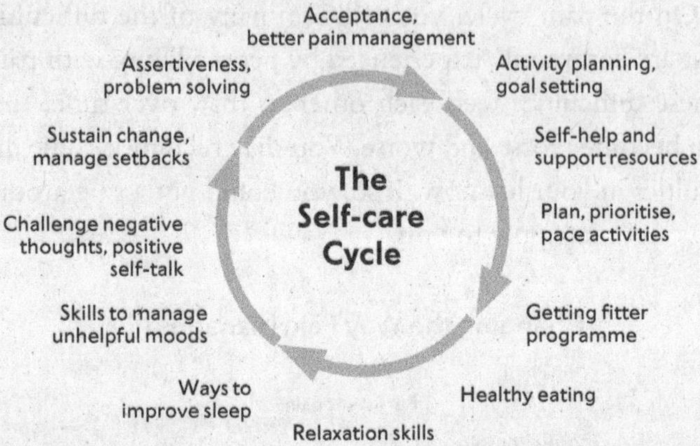

Explore more ideas to start managing pain in the Resources →: page 349.

Ask yourself: what did I learn about changing the impact of pain?

- What I found out.
- What I tried out.
- What went well with my discoveries.

Chapter summary

- Pain affects these five areas of a person: their body (where it causes many symptoms), their moods, their thoughts, their behaviours or actions, and their life situation.
- It is valuable to use the person-centred Five-Areas tool to understand the areas of yourself and your life affected by pain. It helps to see the 'bigger picture' and all the possible positive changes in the five areas.
- It helps to identify two or three issues or needs as priorities to change at one time. These are your targets for change to guide you to ways to manage pain well.
- To start and sustain changes, it can help to:
  - use the Five-Areas tool to help you to work out what things you need to change;
  - be clear about the advantages and disadvantages of making these changes to gain a meaningful life even with pain;
  - give self-management a trial (be willing to explore and experiment; this has helped many people with pain find more rewarding ways of living well);

- get support from others you can trust and notice how things are changing for the better.

Many, many people have learnt how to live a full life with their pain. In time, by exploring the range of skills and tools or resources in this book, you will find this applies to you too.

2

Acceptance and moving on

What this chapter covers

We explore how acceptance can help to manage chronic pain well and confidently. We look at how acceptance can bring more understanding about feelings of loss and grief. We also help you to focus your efforts on becoming the person you would hope to be despite your pain. We will share ways that you can practise being more mindful and aware and actively focused on the present moment. New knowledge about how the brain manages pain suggests that it is important to be kinder, more soothing and more compassionate towards ourselves, a kinder self-awareness.

What is the value of acceptance in managing chronic pain?

Acceptance can help you to live a well and valued life despite your pain and its impact.

When real-life situations do not match expectations, dreams or life-plans, then emotional pain and distress often follow. There is an uncomfortable tricky gap between what was expected, or hoped for, and what is actually happening. And the bigger the gap, the greater the distress or struggle. Acceptance, or willingness to come to terms with your situation, your pain, yourself, can bridge this gap and reduce the emotional pain and discomfort.

To understand this gap that sometimes exists between reality and expectations, let's explore Mo's experiences.

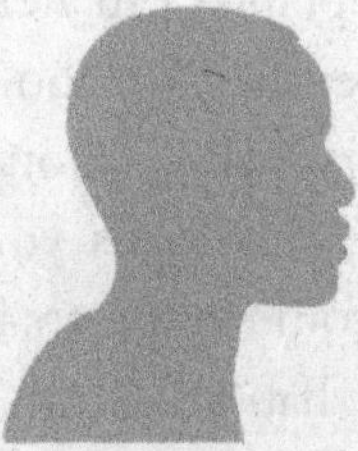

Mo found his neck and shoulder pain got steadily worse over months. Now, two years after his accident, he had given up work and spent most of each day lying on his bed at home. He was sad and fed-up, and asked himself: 'What's the point in anything?' Mo had worked hard in his job as an apprentice. When he stopped work, he felt helpless and unable to change what had happened. Before the accident, he had expected to complete his training and get promotion.

EXPLORING ACCEPTANCE — MO'S EXPERIENCE

The real Mo	THE GAP	The ideal Mo
Who am I now? 'Not the "Mo" who was bright, keen to get on with life' **What's my life like now?** • Cannot work and I so enjoyed the job • Less money/cash • Lost my relationship with Rob, my boyfriend • Spend more time lying in bed in my room • Depressed, sad at what I have lost in two years • Powerless, sometimes defeated		**What did I expect to be doing by now?** • Planned to go to college, have more skills • Be independent and have my own place to live with Rob **What do I think and feel things should be like?** • Happier, travel more, confident to do mountain-biking trails around the country • Hope to go and enjoy music festivals/camping in summer months • Free to do whatever I want

Mo realised there was quite a gap between what he planned and hoped for, and what was truly happening to him.

Now think about your own situation. Is there a gap between your expectations and dreams and your reality? Write down your thoughts, using the questions we've suggested to guide you.

This activity shows the size of the gap at present between your 'real' and 'ideal' ideas about your life. One step towards closing this gap is to be more accepting of where you are in life right now. Other people with pain find that acceptance is a very valuable step to living well with pain. It is tricky to be willing to take the first steps, yet to do so lets you take control of your own journey in life.

Write down your thoughts in answer to the following questions:

EXPLORING ACCEPTANCE

The Real Me	**The Ideal Me**
Who am I now?	What did I expect to be doing at this point in my life?
What is my life like now?	What do I think and feel things should be like?

Understanding more about acceptance

When someone gives you a gift, you may feel excited or happy when you accept it. Trying to accept a situation or event that is unwanted or negative will probably cause you to react very differently indeed. For example, trying to accept that a loved one has died may make someone feel sad, angry and fearful about the future and what might happen now.

One definition of acceptance is: 'experiencing events fully, just as they are and not as they ought to be'. The mindfulness exercises later in this chapter can help you learn how to 'experience events just as they are', without judging them as negative or positive.

Acceptance is not the same as 'giving up' or 'putting your head in the sand'. It is an ongoing journey of change in which people with chronic pain can recognise that their real-life situation is difficult. It may not be what they would have chosen, but they can begin to look at themselves, others, their own thoughts and feelings, and the future in a different, more helpful way.

Acceptance is about grieving and coming to terms with the losses that the pain has brought you and the people in your life, both now and in the future. These changes may be sad and stressful and bring about moods of anger, frustration and perhaps more pain. This vicious cycle does not help the brain to manage pain better.

Unhelpful Cycle of Pain and Non-acceptance

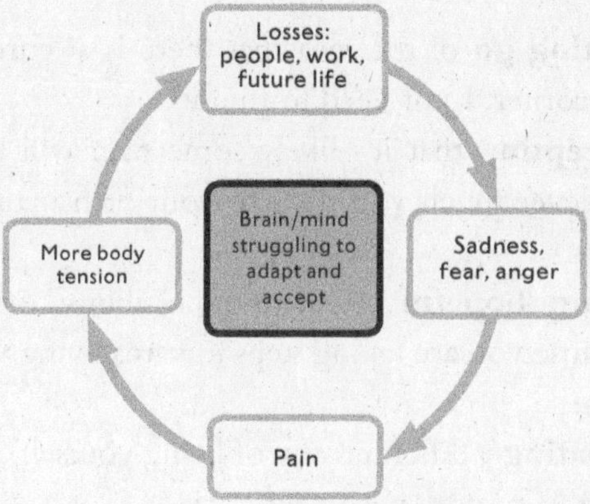

Ultimately, acceptance is about letting go of the 'me without pain' and moving towards accepting that 'I'm still me, just with pain' and creating your own valued self. It is also about true awareness that 'it is not your fault' that pain and hurt have become part of your life and caused much havoc.

This acceptance of your reality can give you a sense of control over your circumstances and your future. It can give you a sense of gratitude for what you do have and a more hopeful and optimistic outlook.

Learning the skills of acceptance

There may be some challenges to work through on the journey towards acceptance, such as:

- **Letting go** of fears and worries about what has been lost.
- **Letting go** of the idea that there is a 'cure around the corner, I just need to find it'.
- **Accepting** that it's likely some pain will be there, however much you stick to your pain management plans.
- **Being hopeful** about the possibility of change, because you are taking steps towards living well with pain.
- **Creating** a different way of being yourself, that lives with pain more positively.

Some people find that it helps to tell themselves: 'I cannot avoid pain, yet I do not have to suffer because of it. ***Pain has wounded me and I can take part in healing myself and a life journey.***'

Changing your outlook on yourself and your future can be hard work and takes both time and being 'willing to let go'. Acceptance is sometimes described as 'a journey', and some people find that spiritual or religious beliefs and teachings can be helpful. For example, some spiritual teachings suggest that humans can experience 'inner healing' without necessarily being 'cured' of their illness or pain.

Having chronic pain may give you an opportunity to look again at what life means to you. It can be about finding a new and *hopeful* meaning in your current life situation. Events that may seem negative can also be seen as openings for growth, interest, a different path or new understanding.

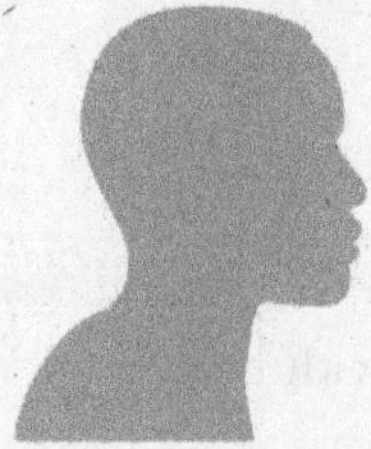

HOW DID MO RESPOND TO THE IDEA OF ACCEPTANCE?

At first, Mo did not expect acceptance to help. He believed it wouldn't change anything really, chiefly the things he had lost in his life.

However, he thought he would take a few steps; as it 'might be worth it, I am willing to give it a try. I am getting stuck in a way of negative thinking of I am useless' and 'life really is not fair to me'. He decided to make some changes. For instance, he talked with his parents about how he could now contribute in the house more. He changed his routine by getting up earlier and using pacing skills so that he could be more active.

However, he still had a lot of pain most days of the week. He realised that, however hard he tried, the pain was still going to be there. At times he was angry about it, but mostly he was sad and found his mind dwelt on his losses.

He talked over the 'meaning of the pain' with Paul, whom he had met at the local health group. Paul helped him to look at the possibilities now that he was at home.

Mo then wrote this list of possibilities for himself now – it took over two hours with help from Paul!

- I was 'there' for my mother after her heart attack.
- I use a digital camera. I've got some great shots of family events recently. Maybe I could make a family album.
- I could train in electronics, so be better qualified.
- I am learning with my mother how to cook on a low budget.
- I have met some fun, caring people in the local self-help group.
- I could help the group develop a website.
- I've been reading more – I never had time for it before. It helps with the forms and letters.
- I've learnt to talk about how I feel, not holding it in and without blaming anyone.
- I realise I am more patient and listen more to others.

Mo was surprised at how many possibilities or benefits he came up with. He said it didn't make up for not being like he used to be. Yet when he thought about the benefits, he realised he felt better and less frustrated.

This is about seeing opportunities or chances rather than focusing on 'making up for the pain'. It is about trying things out and looking to do things another way, even though your current life situation is not what had been planned or expected.

Now think about the opportunities that you have had, or could have, since experiencing chronic pain. They can be small things, not just major ones. Like Mo, you can talk it through with someone if that helps.

Write down five positive changes or new opportunities that have come about since you had chronic pain. Remember that they don't have to be big things – anything counts. If it is more helpful, use a mobile phone or tablet to write your changes.

1. ________________________________

2. ________________________________

3. ________________________________

4. ______________________________

____

____

____

5. ______________________________

____

____

____

____

Techniques to help with acceptance: Mindfulness

Mindfulness is about the kind of awareness that you bring to a situation. It means being in control of what you pay attention to, and for how long. It can be a helpful way of managing distress and many people have learnt to manage their pain more successfully using it. Skills like this are versions of meditation practices taken from Eastern spiritual traditions such as Buddhism. The aim is to be in a 'state of mind' that is more helpful to manage and live well with pain. This state of mind helps the brain to process pain in helpful ways, and is soothing and calming.

How can mindfulness help?

When you focus on your pain, it can lead to distress and unhelpful negative thinking about yourself and the future. This increases tension within your body and leads to more worrying or anxious thoughts. Finding different ways of using your awareness – for example by practising relaxed breathing, without becoming distressed – can really help manage pain. In turn, this can change the way that you experience the pain.

Unhelpful Cycle of Pain and Non-acceptance

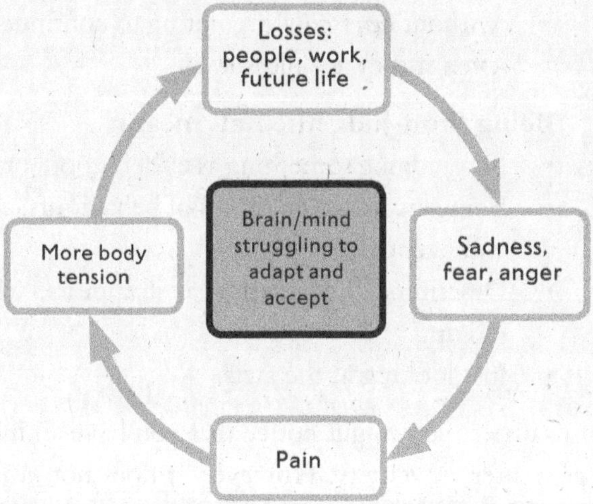

Mindfulness aims to balance ‘reasonable’ and ‘emotional’ thinking. It uses a ‘wise mind’ thinking approach to being with yourself as you are and your life in the now.

Mindfulness skills

These are four main mindfulness skills: observing, being 'non-judgemental', focusing on one thing now, and doing what works.

1. **Observing practice means** paying attention to events, emotions and behaviours:
   - without *necessarily* attempting to stop them even if they are painful;
   - without *necessarily* attempting to continue them even if they are pleasurable.

2. **Being 'non-judgemental' means:**
   - Not judging something as either 'good' or 'bad'.
   - Being aware of the results of behaviours, actions and events.
   - Describing the situation as it appears, without judging.
   - Just looking at the facts.

   For example, you might notice that you have an increase in pain after an activity. However, it does not *necessarily* mean the outcome is 'bad'. It does not necessarily mean it is 'good' either. It is just some 'more pain'.

3. **Focusing on one thing now and being in the present moment means:**
   - Guiding your attention and actively focusing

on your senses – what you hear, see, smell, taste and so on.

- Noticing memories of the past or worries about the future, yet not becoming distracted by them.
- Noticing negative moods or thoughts, yet re-focusing the mind into the present moment. This means moods and thoughts distract you less.

It is possible to learn to focus attention on one task or activity at a time. It does take practice. Being gentle and supportive with yourself helps as you experiment and discover.

4. **Doing activities and what helps change for you:**
   - Focusing on the goals you set yourself.
   - Realising that what works well for a person or a situation may not work for another, so shaping your own 'self'.
   - Understanding that what used to work before, may not work now.
   - Realising that doing what you 'ought' to do may not work for you in the present time (e.g. being the sole breadwinner, making sure all washing and ironing is done every day, etc.).
   - Taking people as they are, rather than as you might think they 'should' be (including yourself)!

Mindfulness exercises

Here are some exercises that you can do to experiment with attentional control or mindfulness.

A mindful breathing exercise

- Give yourself a few minutes to sit quietly.
- Notice your breathing.
- Pay attention to your breath going in and coming out.
- Try to let your attention focus on the bottom of your in-breath.
- Actively 'let go' as you breathe out.
- When you notice that your thoughts have wandered, always bring your attention back to your breathing.
- Spend a few minutes bringing your attention back to the centre in this way.

This can lead to a state of feeling calm and secure.

A mindful observation exercise

- Be aware of your hand on a cool surface (e.g. a table or a glass of cold water). Be aware of your hand on a warm surface (e.g. your other hand).
- Pay attention to, and try to sense, your stomach and your shoulders.
- Stroke just above your upper lip. Stop stroking.

Notice how long it takes before you cannot sense your upper lip any longer.

- 'Watch' the first two thoughts that come into your mind – just **notice** them.
- Imagine that your mind is a conveyor belt and that thoughts and feelings are coming down the belt. Put each thought or feeling in a box near the belt.
- Count the thoughts or feelings as you have them.
- If you find yourself becoming distracted, observe that too. Observe yourself, as you notice that you are being distracted.

Note: It is usual to have to start and re-start several times when you practise 'stepping back' and observing in this way.

A 'describing', 'non-judgemental' exercise

- Practise labelling thoughts in groups, such as 'thoughts about others' or 'thoughts about myself'.
- Use the 'conveyor belt' exercise described above. As the thoughts and feelings come down the conveyor belt, imagine sorting them into boxes, e.g. one box for thoughts, one box for sensations in your body, one for urges to do something, etc.

Make a point of practising **most often** the exercises that you find most difficult.

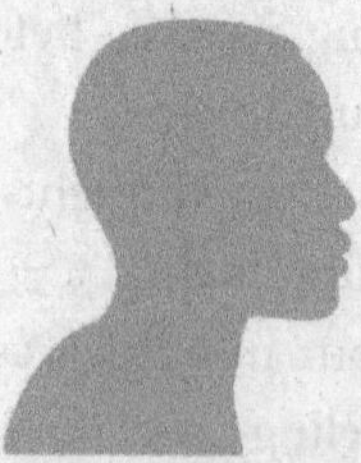

Mo found out more from Paul about a mindfulness group and decided to try it. He tried the mindful breathing practice and found that his mind wandered a lot. It filled with thoughts about how his life was or just everyday things. He learnt to gently guide his mind back to focus on his breathing without getting cross about it. He learnt to observe what his mind or body did without reacting or judging it or being critical. After the fourth session, he became aware of times when his mind seemed calmer and other times when it was quite stressed. He realised that when he was stressed, he hurt more. Then, when his mind was calm, he found he was struggling less as 'it is only the pain as it usually is, nothing dangerous', so the pain experience seems less.

He used a mindful app, which Paul suggested, so he could practise most days.

He experimented with mindful movement exercises too and found how to move more easily and gently with his breathing as the focus. He found his body relaxed and soothed; some of his pain dissolved and he was more flexible in his back. 'I don't feel so frightened and now

I see how to help the brain turn down the pain intensity and sensitivity' →: page 66.

All these mindful activities will give an insight into the level of control over what you focus your attention on.

With regular practice, these skills can:

- reduce the amount of time you are distracted by your pain;
- reduce your mind's constant struggle with pain so you feel less stressed.

Daily practice means you will find it easier to deliberately pay attention to something else more valued. This, in turn, will help you 'accept the things you cannot change', and 'change the things you can'. Mindfulness helps both reduce adrenaline chemicals in the body that wind up pain intensity and sensitivity, and release the brain's own opioids to soothe, calm, control pain and lessen suffering or hurt.

Explore Resources →: page 357 to guide your exploration of acceptance and self-compassion; and what they mean and ways they can help.

Chapter summary

What did I value from this chapter?

Tick what you valued and/or that helped in becoming more accepting of chronic pain.

- ❑ Acceptance is an important part of learning to live well with chronic pain and other health conditions.
- ❑ When losses have occurred, it is essential to:
    - allow time to get used to what has happened;
    - allow yourself to grieve for what has been lost;
    - learn how to cope with what is happening 'here and now'.
- ❑ It can help to find 'meaning' in what has happened and practise noticing unexpected opportunities.
- ❑ Mindful attention helps focus on areas and priorities of your life in which to invest change rather than being involved with the mindless distraction of pain.
- ❑ Your own values and view of the world can make it easier for you to cope with long-term

difficulties. Some people find that spiritual practice or meditation can help.

- ❑ Mindfulness exercises are a useful regular practice to reduce suffering and distress with the struggle to be rid of pain. They can help manage pain and enable you to live well without giving up or losing hope.
- ❑ Other things I valued about this chapter . . .

____

____

____

____

3

Knowing more about pain and the brain

Discover more about pain, the brain and the body

The focus of this chapter is understanding why we have pain. It explores how the brain and the nerve network system create and manage pain. It covers the different types of pain and we look at acute (short-term) and chronic (long-term) pain. Research over the last ten years has enabled pain scientists to understand much more about how the brain and nervous system create pain. This knowledge helps provide a map and a vision for the future about possible ways that pain might be relieved or managed.

What is pain?

A worldwide group of pain specialists (International Association for the Study of Pain (IASP)) in 1979 defined pain as:

An unpleasant sensory and emotional experience which is due to actual or potential tissue damage or which is expressed in terms of such damage.

This is the definition most doctors and other health professionals use when assessing pain, including **your** pain. Recently, the understanding of pain has changed a lot. Doctors, nurses, physiotherapists and other healthcare professionals **used** to think:

- that pain systems in the body are very simple; ***and***
- if you can find the cause of the acute pain problem/s you can 'fix it'; ***and***
- the best way to manage acute pain is to rest and then, as healing starts, slowly to get active, which helps with healing and keeps the body fitter and healthy.

Now healthcare professionals know:

- that resting only for a few days before starting to get active again helps acute or 'short-term pain'; ***and***
- that if you have chronic pain, rest is usually unhelpful and often makes the pain experience worse.

Why is chronic pain different from acute pain?

Research into pain shows that ***chronic pain is very different to acute pain*** and trying to 'fix it' with drugs or treatments usually fails.

It turns out that the experience of pain is very complicated. It relies on the way the brain, spinal cord and the nervous system or nerve networks interact with each other.

→ : See diagram opposite.

Understanding more about different types of pain shows that the treatment or management of chronic pain needs a different approach from that of acute pain. Sadly, chronic pain itself cannot be cured or fixed yet. Changing the approach from trying to 'fix or sort the chronic pain' to 'manage it better' helps reduce some of the distress and suffering, and some of the pain experience itself.

The year 2019 saw a real milestone in managing chronic pain when the World Health Organisation and the International Association for the Study of Pain agreed to include chronic pain and the different types of chronic pain in the system that classifies diseases ICD 11[1] and which will be used in healthcare systems from 2022 across the globe. This important international step recognises that chronic pain is a disease, with many unhelpful changes in the brain and nerve network systems. This type of pain requires a person-centred Five-Areas multi-focused approach on managing distressing body symptoms, moods difficulties, life stresses and unhelpful behaviours. It also means better research and more data about pain, as it will be easier to record information about types of pain. The ICD-11 data entry system will make it easier to record information about pain types and areas, so guide better ways to manage it.

1 International Classification of Disease = ICD version 11.

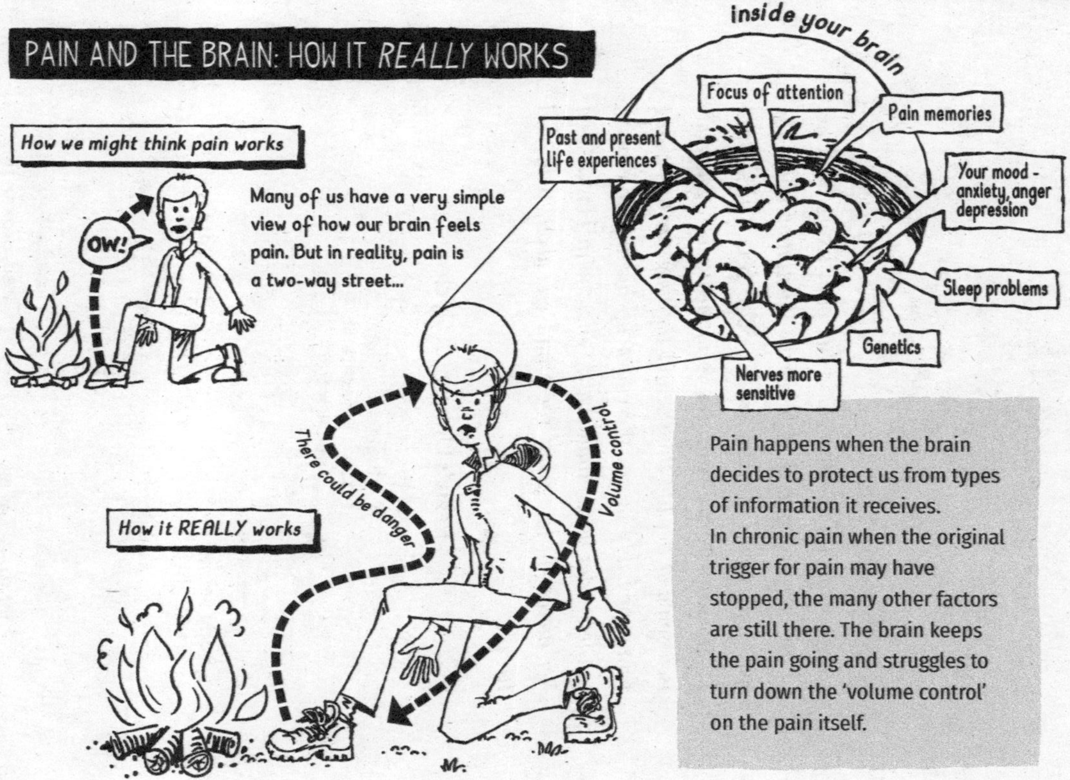
PAIN AND THE BRAIN: HOW IT *REALLY* WORKS
How we might think pain works
OW!
Many of us have a very simple view of how our brain feels pain. But in reality, pain is a two-way street...
How it REALLY works
There could be danger
Volume control
inside your brain
Past and present life experiences
Focus of attention
Pain memories
Your mood - anxiety, anger depression
Sleep problems
Genetics
Nerves more sensitive
Pain happens when the brain decides to protect us from types of information it receives.
In chronic pain when the original trigger for pain may have stopped, the many other factors are still there. The brain keeps the pain going and struggles to turn down the 'volume control' on the pain itself.

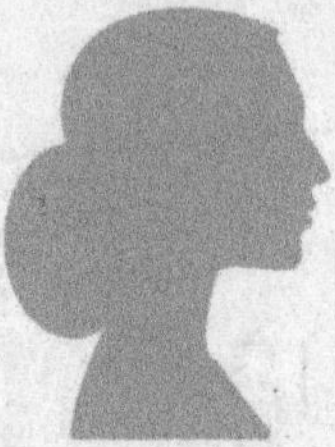

Razia struggled to understand her pain issues, and her physiotherapist shared with her the illustration about the way brain handles pain. →: page 55. *This helped Razia see why the pain was so unpredictable. She realised some of her life stresses and the way she was doing things probably meant she ended up having more pain, not less! Her next hurdle was to share with Hassan and her mother-in-law what she found out about pain and its role.*

Razia's Unhelpful Cycle

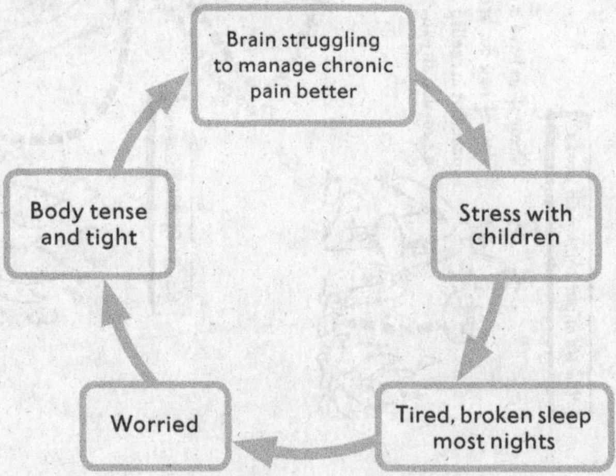

Thinking about your pain

Chronic pain problems are very common. As many as one in five people are affected by chronic pain, often in different parts of their bodies. Pain is a very personal experience and only you really know how your own pain feels. It can be difficult to find the words to describe it to other people. This can make it hard for them to understand how distressed your pain makes you feel, and how it affects the way you think and react.

Think about how you would describe your pain to someone. For instance, you might use words that describe the **pain sensation**, such as 'sharp', 'shooting', 'nagging' or 'aching'. Or you might use words to describe how it **makes you feel**, such as 'worried', 'scared', 'angry', 'down', 'guilty' or 'fed-up'.

You might describe what you **think or believe** about your pain, such as:

- I knew I shouldn't have lifted that heavy container at work.
- Pain means I've been injured. It hurts, so I shouldn't move the pain area until it goes away.

- Headaches run in my family. I knew I would get them at some time in my life.
- Bad backs never get better.
- It's a damaged nerve after the shingles. It must be serious!

Looking at how the pain affects you physically or limits you, what activities or behaviours have you **stopped** or do you now **do differently**?

Explore Maria's example and then try with your own pain experiences using the Five-Areas tool.

Here, in Maria's Five-Areas tool, she is describing the effect of pain on her activities and behaviours. She added some more things, too, to describe her pain, like tired and sleeping poorly.

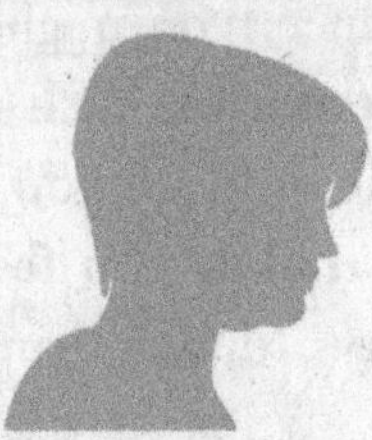

Maria

I cannot bend and pick things up from the floor.
It alters the way I move – I walk so stiffly.
The pain makes me lie down more often.
It stops me going out with friends.
I feel fed-up about it . . . it is more than I thought!

Maria's Pain Experience Using Five-Areas Tool

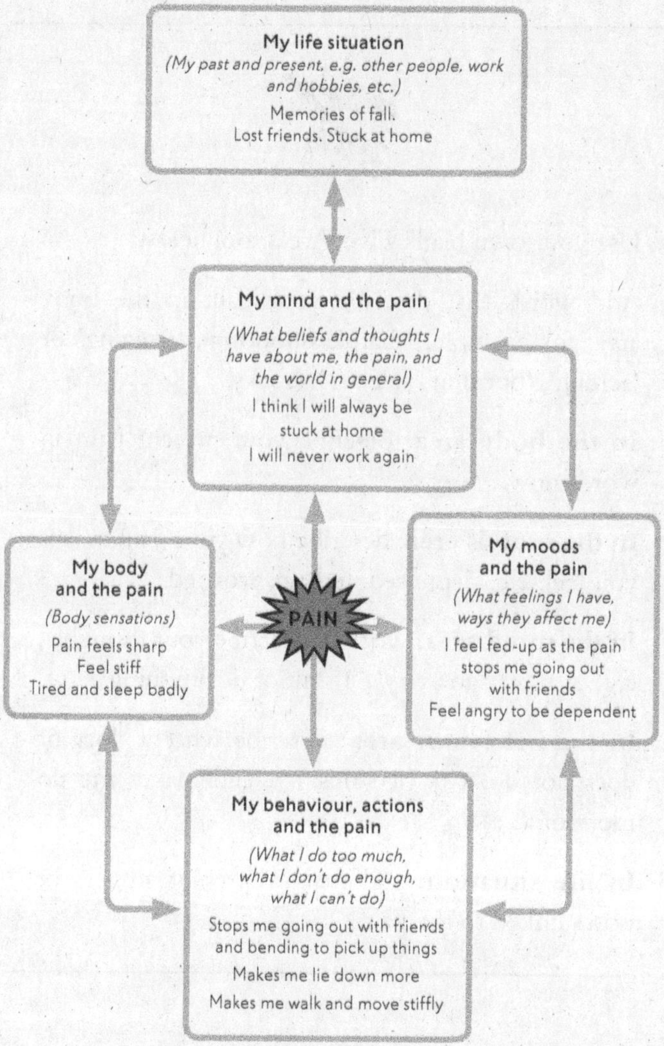

My life situation
(My past and present, e.g. other people, work and hobbies, etc.)
Memories of fall.
Lost friends. Stuck at home
My mind and the pain
(What beliefs and thoughts I have about me, the pain, and the world in general)
I think I will always be stuck at home
I will never work again
My body and the pain
(Body sensations)
Pain feels sharp
Feel stiff
Tired and sleep badly
PAIN
My moods and the pain
(What feelings I have, ways they affect me)
I feel fed-up as the pain stops me going out with friends
Feel angry to be dependent
My behaviour, actions and the pain
(What I do too much, what I don't do enough, what I can't do)
Stops me going out with friends and bending to pick up things
Makes me lie down more
Makes me walk and move stiffly

Now let's explore further your pain.

Use your own blank Five-Areas tool below:

Add words that describe your pain in the body area; for example, 'sharp', 'shooting', 'nagging' or 'aching', 'burning', 'electric shocks'.

In the body area: describe your present pain in words now.

In the moods area: describe how your pain makes you feel, e.g. depressed, fed-up, worried.

In the mind area: write or describe your thoughts, e.g. 'it won't go away', 'I cannot do anything'.

In the behaviour area: describe what it does or does not do, e.g. 'it stops . . . and makes me do more of . . .'

In life situation: add past or present stresses or issues linked to the pain.

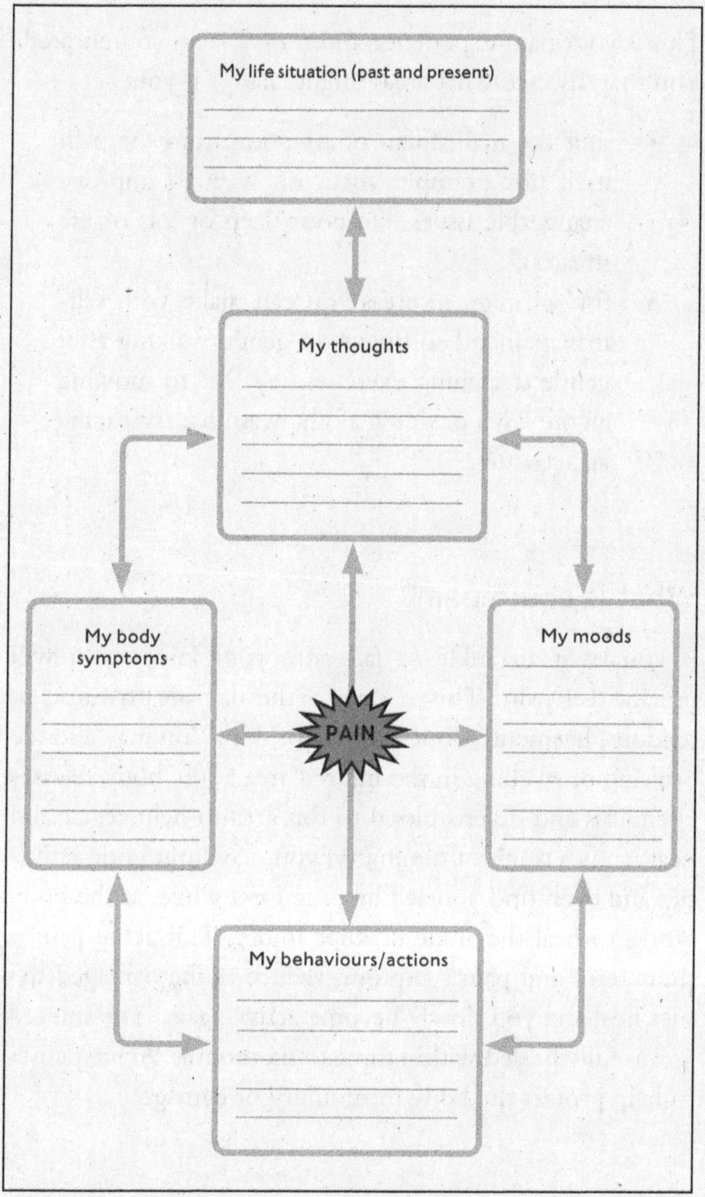
My life situation (past and present)
My thoughts
My body symptoms
PAIN
My moods
My behaviours/actions

This is your pain experience and it may seem complicated. You may also see what areas might change if you:

- shift the main focus of attention from the pain itself (for example, focus on ways to improve changeable issues like poor sleep or lots of life stresses);
- find changes in areas you can make with self-management; so, focus on gentle walking after gentle stretching exercises, say 'no' to mowing all the lawn or doing all the washing; try pacing all activities.

What is acute pain?

If you twist an ankle or fall onto your knees, you will usually feel pain. This is due to the damage to muscles, tendons, ligaments, bones, nerves or skin. You may also see bruising or swelling in the injured area as the body releases chemicals and diverts blood to this area to help repair and heal it. As a result of the injury, you may limit your activities and even find yourself limping for a while, as the body works to heal the ankle or knee injury. This acute pain is short term and pain symptoms reduce as the damaged tissues heal and you slowly become active again. The injured area is fully healed within three to six months. Acute pain is to help protect the body from injury or damage.

What is chronic pain?

This is pain that continues for longer than three to six months. It does not reduce or disappear even when muscles, ligaments, broken bones or nerves are healed, and it may even get worse.

Research into chronic pain shows that the real problems exist in the nerve networks and their message systems that communicate between the body and the brain and spinal cord – the central nervous system.

Explore the pain puzzles below – they show that to understand pain better, we need to know how the brain interprets what is felt and seen.

PAIN PUZZLES FOR ACUTE AND CHRONIC PAIN

Acute Pain Puzzle: Some athletes injured in sports events, or soldiers injured in battle, do not notice or feel pain at the time they are injured, even when the injury is very large.

Why is this? *There is a shift in focus of attention in the brain; for example, the soldier is totally focused on survival at the point of injury.*

Acute Pain Puzzle: A person wearing boots has trodden on a sharp nail. It looks like the nail has gone directly into the foot itself. An X-ray of the foot shows that the nail has gone through the boot, between the toes and not entered into the foot all. Yet the person was in great pain and distress.

Why is this? *The person was in severe pain because* ***he/she thought*** *it had gone through the boot and into the foot itself. In other words, the brain has interpreted what it saw incorrectly. It believed a serious injury had happened because it saw the nail had gone through the boot and jumped to the conclusion into the foot itself.*

Chronic Pain Puzzle: People who have had a limb – for example, a leg – removed can still experience pain in it years later. This is called 'phantom limb pain'.

Why is this? *Memories of the limb and pain are encoded or programmed into the brain's memory systems. Also, the nerve network and its sensors are more sensitive.*

These puzzles show that the body's pain systems are much more complex than people realise. They show that pain can be linked to the personal meaning of an event or situation or other factors.

What we know about acute pain

The role of acute pain is to keep us safe and protect us from further harm or damage.

The body has nerve fibre endings called sensors to detect heat, touch, pressure, movement and other changes. These nerve fibre sensors help detect changes that may indicate damage, injury or threat to the body. For example, if you lift a hot pan from a stove or sip a very hot drink, the heat sensors pick up the real possibility of heat damage to your hand or mouth. The brain produces pain in your hands or mouth, as they are at risk of the danger of burn damage. This warns you to stop what you are doing immediately, to prevent damage. The brain reacts to the sensors extremely quickly and gets you to:

- stop sipping the hot drink to stop any damage to the mouth or gullet, as this would be dangerous;
- let go of the pan to avoid your hand being burnt by the pan's heat.

How does it happen?

Heat sensors in the skin or lips notice the *dangerous* level of heat and send messages very fast, through the spinal cord nerve networks, to the brain. The brain assesses and responds to keep you safe. It stops you drinking or makes your hand move immediately from the *dangerous* heat source to stop burning yourself. →: See 'pain and the brain' illustration on page 55.

Acute pain is a key survival system designed to protect the body and the brain. It may help to compare it to dialling straight through to the emergency services so that action is taken to respond to the serious or life-threatening incident.

What we understand about chronic pain

Acute pain is what we feel when the sensors, nerve networks and brain system are working together to keep us from danger/harm. This is not the case with chronic pain; it is **different**. We now understand that there are problems in all these three areas in chronic pain; so, the

1. **nerve fibre sensors** pick up changes in temperature or touch/pressure or other sensations or movements;
2. **nerve networks** then communicate those changes from the body areas to the brain system to process;
3. way the **brain system** assesses and processes the changes and then makes decisions on the action needed to deal with the 'painful' threat.

Some of these problems we understand; others need more knowledge and so much more research.

1. Change in nerve fibre sensor sensitivity

The nerve fibre sensors in the body that detect changes

in heat, touch, pressure and so on can become over-sensitive and over-react. So, the sensors produce many more messages than they need to. The brain interprets these incoming messages as possible or probable danger in that body area, even if it is already healed or repaired. This increased sensitivity confuses the brain. It struggles to block out or ignore all the inaccurate information it gets from these sensors. The sensitivity change is due to many chemical changes within the sensors themselves. We don't yet know about what continues to trigger these changes or what stops them.

It may help to think of the sensor reactions as similar to those in a burglar alarm system. Here, an alarm sensor picks up movement change to indicate the possible presence of a human being, possibly a burglar. If the sensor becomes more sensitive, it will pick up smaller changes in movement and trigger the alarm system more often, unhelpfully and inaccurately.

2. Problems with nerve fibre sensors and nerve networks and pain

Three main problems are common: sensors become over-sensitive, memory of pain happens in the nerve fibres, nerve fibres can be physically damaged.

a. These sensors continue over months and years to become very sensitive to movement, hot and cold sensations, and chemical changes (such as inflammation from injury, infections or medications within the body). Sometimes if the painful area is touched or moved, the sensors send more and more pointless messages to the brain. This magnifies the sensations so the brain interprets them as dangerous even though nothing is actually wrong at all. The result is more pain. Often, other sensations like numbness or tingling are added in. This process is now called central sensitisation of the sensor – nerve – brain networks.

b. Some nerve fibres develop a 'memory' of body sensation or pain experiences. They continue to send danger messages for many months or years after an injury, even when healing is completed. These fibres are like a set of traffic lights stuck on red that cannot switch itself back to green. *Phantom limb pain* is an example.

c. The nerve network wiring or fibres can also be damaged, causing over-sensitive sensors and more pain. This can happen when nerves get accidentally crushed or after a burn or chemical injury and is called *neuropathic pain*. An example is shingles, a virus infection of the nerve fibre itself. This infection can damage the nerve 'wiring' structure so that it remains over-sensitive and/or over-reactive to everyday activities such as moving about or wearing clothing in the shingles infection area. This sensitivity is known as *neuralgia*, meaning a painful sensitive nerve, and is a type of neuropathic pain.

3. Problems with the brain assessing information

The brain has a challenging job to do when it receives information of danger or harm.

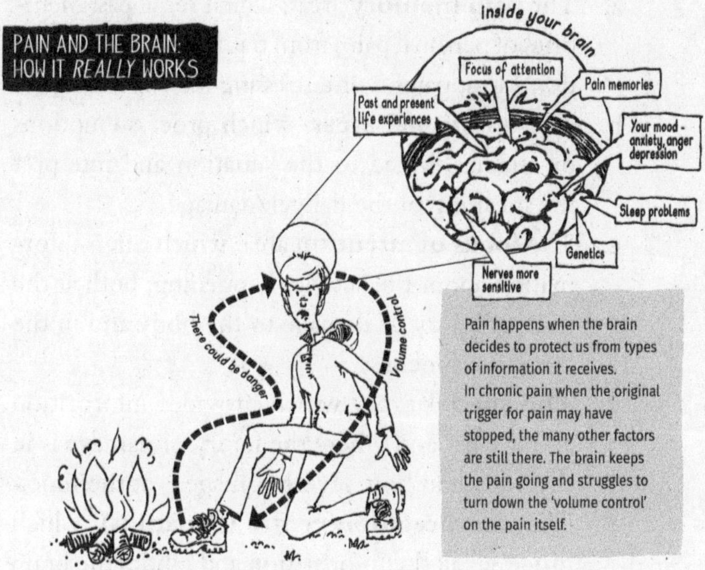
PAIN AND THE BRAIN:
HOW IT *REALLY* WORKS
Inside your brain
Focus of attention
Pain memories
Past and present life experiences
Your mood - anxiety, anger depression
Sleep problems
Genetics
Nerves more sensitive
There could be danger
Volume control
Pain happens when the brain decides to protect us from types of information it receives.
In chronic pain when the original trigger for pain may have stopped, the many other factors are still there. The brain keeps the pain going and struggles to turn down the 'volume control' on the pain itself.

It needs to process and assess all the information it constantly receives from different areas or centres in the body. It then needs to know what it should do to help the body to take action to keep safe. Some areas in the brain like the memory and emotional areas (that generate anxiety, anger and other moods) can react very quickly, and this leads to more misinterpretation or confusion in assessing pain. There are many areas that receive information within the brain about the specific situation; some are:

a. The **pain memory** areas, which recall past memories of personal pain, from trauma or injury, emotional loss, painful or distressing life experiences.
b. The **emotional areas**, which process emotions or feelings linked to the situation and interpret the meaning of the danger/damage.
c. The **focus of attention** area, which offers information about the activity happening, both at the time of injury or damage to the body and in the current moment.
d. **The spatial area**, which provides information about what and where the injury or damage is in the body and how severe damage is at the time.
e. The **interpretation centre (thalamus)**, which processes all the information and guides the brain on what action to tell the body to take. This is similar to air traffic control guiding air flights in and out of airports safely. If there is a lot of emotional feeling and traumatic memories linked to pain, then it is as if all the planes are arriving to land at the airport at one time: pretty dangerous!
f. **Human genetic data**, which has programmed the brain to be aware of key sensations that indicate life-threatening danger. For example, the brain is already programmed by our gene

information to identify that animal stings may be harmful, such as a scorpion sting or a bite from a deadly snake. Therefore, when we experience a sharp pin-prick sensation on the skin, we can react as if we've actually been stung by a dangerous life-threatening animal not a more friendly, curious and harmless insect, such as the spider rather than the scorpion.

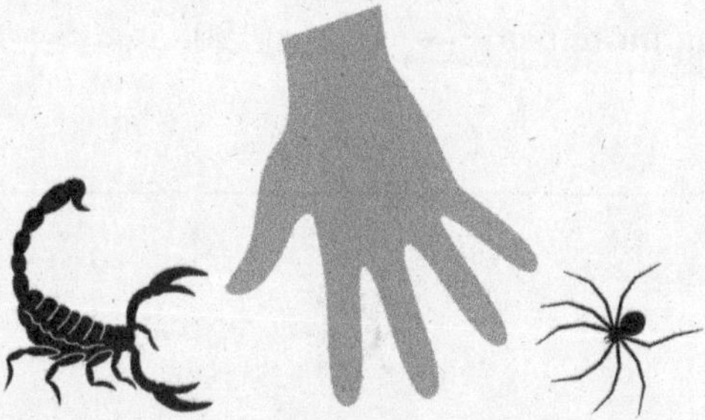

The brain processes and assesses all this information, and in chronic pain makes a decision that there is danger. It produces pain, yet there is no danger and the body itself is safe.

The processing and assessment of lots of information that indicates danger can mean:

1. the brain struggles or fails to make sense of all the different information it receives;
2. it is less able to block off or reduce the numbers of many different incoming signals of possible danger;
3. it continues to interpret continuing sensor messages

as meaning the pain problem is still happening and the body area is not healed.

The result is chronic pain.

Then all these changes worsen when we are tired, frustrated, stressed. Lots of research shows that poor sleep patterns are common for people with chronic pain. Poor sleep and tiredness change the way the brain processes information into these unhelpful ways, which may result in you feeling more pain →: page 190.

> Explore more about Pain and the Brain with the online resources suggested in Resources (→: page 349) for helpful explanations that include 'Understanding pain in five minutes': https://www.youtube.com/watch?v=5KrUL8tOaQs.

How can this help you to manage chronic pain?

It is crucial to know that some reasons for chronic pain are changeable, as Mo found out.

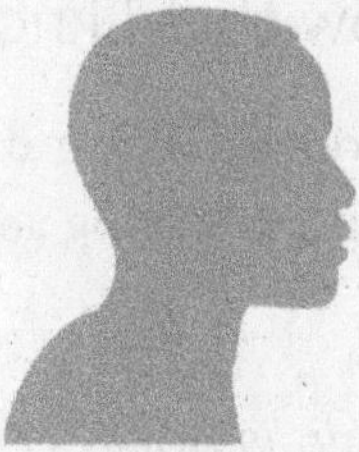

Mo's story

Mo had not understood after his motorbike accident about types of pain. He explored the above YouTube video titled 'Understanding pain in five minutes'. He realised that:

- *the healed scar tissue becomes tight, stiff, less flexible;*
- *the nerves themselves can be wrapped up within this scar tissue and so nerves can become more sensitive;*
- *so when moving these parts of the body, many more danger messages occur. The brain misinterprets these messages and believes this is probably harmful, so pain persists.*

Mo had stopped his activities and rested up. This actually made his pain experience worse. His brain got stuck on believing the painful injury damage was still there, when in fact it had healed leaving the affected areas tight, stiff, weak and unfit. 'I thought you had to rest up with pain and it would go; it seemed the natural thing to do. Sometimes just thinking about moving hurts! Now I get it; I am getting fitter . . . and more positive too. I wish I had known this months ago.'

What can I do now that I know more?

Explore the chapters on Balancing daily activities through pacing and Being fitter and staying active → : page 150.

1. Recognise the brain is not 100 per cent reliable

The way that the brain processes information from the nerve networks and sensors means that the body is not always a reliable guide when it comes to chronic pain. Sometimes, some of the pain can come from several causes, as Mo discovered, and these are changeable. Being aware of this will help you to become a better manager of your pain.

Very often, people with pain become fearful of moving certain parts of the body because they think it will cause more harm and more pain. When they discover that their experiences of pain may be unreliable and based on faulty information, this new awareness allows them to find ways of moving more, getting stronger and achieving more control over their pain.

2. Change how you think about pain

Help the brain to realise it is safe to move and be active. It seems that if you help the brain to understand that there is no more damage or injury happening, it makes better sense of the situation. The brain can change its own nerve networks activity, a process called neuroplasticity. This means that the brain is able to change how it receives and processes information to create nerve networks that respond in more useful ways. In other words, become a more reliable interpreter of information. Practically, this means changing the meaning of the pain you feel; for example, from 'It hurts when I move so there must be something wrong or damaged' to saying to yourself and your brain, 'It hurts when I move as the muscles are tight and stiff. It will help if I build up my fitness steadily, so less pain.'

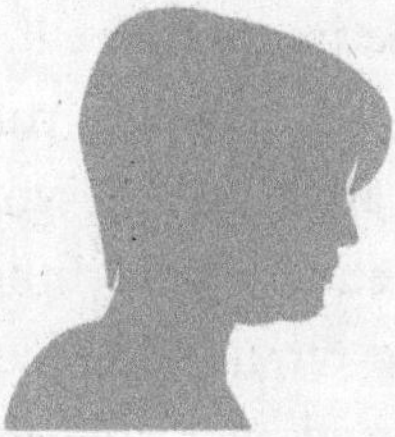

Maria was worried that bending forward might cause damage in her bones and lead to tearing of her muscles. The result was that her back became very stiff, which caused more pain and disability. She learnt more about pain and the brain from her physio, and realised that gentle stretches helped her back. She understood how her fears of causing more damage were inaccurate and a misinterpretation.

It is very common for people with pain to become fearful of moving certain parts of the body because they think it will cause more harm and more pain. When they discover that their experiences of pain may be unreliable and based on faulty information, this new awareness allows them to find ways of moving more, getting stronger and achieving greater control over their pain.

3. Move more often

Increasing flexibility in stiff, tight tissues, like scars, muscles and so on, may reduce the pain and its effects. Changes like regular gradual body stretching and strengthening help the nerve fibres to become less sensitive to movement. Like Mo, you may want to experiment to see if, over several weeks as you get more active, you have less pain as you retrain your brain. Options like t'ai chi, gentle yoga and other mindful movement, balance and healthy fitness programmes help the brain readjust and retrain. The neuroplastic changes in the brain can be reversed over time and the nerves, muscle, etc. become less reactive and sensitive to movement.

4. Kind self-care actions

These can make a difference, so spot your unhelpful behaviours and make changes. Jim had unhelpful pacing in the following example.

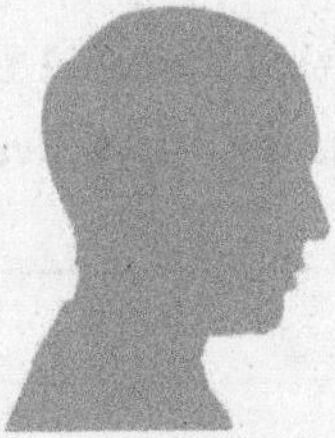

Jim struggles to pace his day's activities well. He overdoes activity and exercise in a 'boom and bust pattern', as he tends to believe that the activity 'must' be completed even if in severe pain.

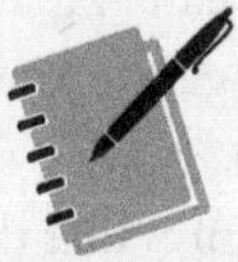

Circle below Jim's wind-up stresses to his brain and what causes his pain levels to increase

tiredness

restless sleep

muscle cramps

lists of things to do

worry

watch a fun movie

more coffee to keep going

What might wind down these stresses to the brain?

Check the self-care cycle → : page 28 and make some suggestions to guide him.

What helpful actions could I do or change to wind down stresses to my brain?

___

___

___

Some things like worry and pressured thinking tire Jim, both his brain and body, and mean his pain levels can increase. Changing to balancing activities through the day, along with relaxation or gentle stretches, enables Jim's brain to be more aware that the body is safe and in balance. It also means there are less pressures that threaten it too. Being kind in this way to both the body and brain helps them be less sensitive and over-reactive. It may actually help the brain to produce more soothing natural opioids, called endorphins, that help lessen pain and upset.

'Looking after me, too, really helps,' was Jim's conclusion after a month of balanced pacing of activities, drinking less coffee and gentle relaxation breaks, some with music. 'Keeping it up is my next challenge.'

The development of self-care skills like goal setting, pacing and getting fitter, among others, really help the brain rebalance itself and manage pain better.

5. Kind and soothing positive self-talk

Share with yourself that you are coping well with activities in the day despite the pain levels. This will guide your brain to interpret the situations and pain more accurately. This in turn lessens stress and the release of adrenaline, which 'winds up' the pain networks and stimulates more pain. It seems the brain and nerve networks really benefit from 'well-being' thinking to pain and health issues → : page 341.

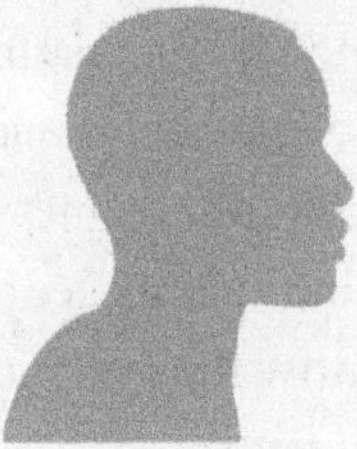

Mo started to tell himself that his neck, shoulder and knee healed well and that gentle stretches made him more flexible. Some of the pains he felt were just stiffness or tight hamstring muscles from so much sitting or lying around. He realised his body hurt more as it was tight and unfit, and maybe it would help to include more stretching exercises and gently build fitness. After six weeks he was amazed at how far he could pace his walking by taking breaks and telling himself, 'Of course it hurts a bit; this is normal when I am stretching and rebuilding my fitness; the pain seems thirty per cent less than when I started. I can now walk to and from the local shops, about one kilometre. I feel my confidence is up, maybe thirty-five per cent.'

Chapter summary

What did you learn from this chapter? Tick below in the summary box.

- ❑ Acute pain and chronic pain are different types of pain and need to be managed differently.
- ❑ The brain and nerve network systems are complicated, and pain scientists and healthcare professionals now understand that chronic pain is not curable, yet.
- ❑ The brain struggles to interpret incoming information accurately 100 per cent of the time in chronic pain.
- ❑ Sensors communicate danger or harm to the body and are over-sensitive in chronic pain.
- ❑ The brain and nerve system are changeable (or neuroplastic), so it is possible to help the brain manage pain better.
- ❑ A balanced healthy approach to using a range of self-care skills like pacing, setting realistic goals, getting fitter, ways to sleep well and positive self-talk are some of the useful skills to cultivate.

- ❑ It helps to be both kind to yourself in thinking and actions and more accepting that chronic pain is not 'fixable'. This helps the brain to feel safe, soothed and less over-reactive.
- ❑ Other things I found out, such as suggested online resources to explore.

4

Support for self-management

What this chapter covers

In this chapter we explore the role of different healthcare professionals and working together with them, so you can get the best from their support to live well in spite of pain.

We will look at knowing more about what they do and what to expect from them, along with ideas on ways to make the most of their support. There is information about pain management programme group work, and talking therapies that can help build your confidence and skills in living well with pain.

Healthcare professionals are clinicians who have had specific clinical training and been assessed to practise or licensed to practise via their professional title and organisation. Their organisation ensures that the expected standards and quality of care are delivered, and failure to provide these can lead to removal of their licence to practise.

Why healthcare professionals can help

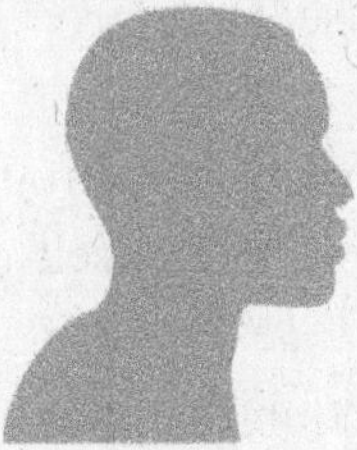

Mo's boyfriend Rob was tired of hearing about Mo's pain. Mo just talked about all the things that he couldn't do any more. Rob could see that the pain was in control of Mo's life. When Rob started college, Mo realised that he would hold Rob back if he didn't start doing things differently, adapting and building new skills. Mo talked about his limitations with his physio during his second session. The latter suggested that maybe it was time to look at dealing with pain in different ways. Mo was curious to know more.

Like many people with chronic pain, Mo found that both pain and how it affected him controlled much of his life. You may have discovered this as well when you used the pain cycle in Maria's story ➔: page 27. Mo found it was helpful to share with his physiotherapist how pain controlled his day-to-day life. This was a step in the right direction, as he began to see the value of specific healthcare professional support. It offered a valuable step to guide his changes and build his confidence in managing pain. Working closely, learning and doing experiments with the support of healthcare professionals can help you to make positive changes. They help you to look at:

- pain and its management through a different way of thinking, often using the self-care cycle as a starter guide; and to
- plan with you action that you might take to improve things without increasing your pain.

See ➔: page 28.

Useful things to know: who healthcare professionals are and what they can do

Pain probably affects you in different ways, so a range of skills and expertise are needed at different times. Sometimes two or more healthcare professionals will work with you at one time.

Currently, do you have support from a health-care professional?

Circle the professionals working with you at present

General practitioner Nurse practitioner

Psychologist Cognitive behavioural therapist

Pain specialist physiotherapist

Pain specialist nurse

Pain medicine specialist Pharmacist

Other None

Understanding the different roles of these professionals to help you manage pain, and working closely with them to benefit from their expert experience and skills, can be extremely valuable in meeting your needs.

Where services are available, these healthcare professionals will have extensive training in their own special clinical area and be very experienced in working with person-centred approaches in many aspects of pain management.

Other healthcare professionals, such as your general practitioner or family physician, are not specialists in pain management. They have a general range of healthcare skills to help you identify and deal with some of your needs and point you to other self-management services.

This summary table shows the different skills and support that each health professional group can offer to guide your self-management.

Looking at the table summary on the next page, can you see why Mo chose to work with a physiotherapist or physical therapist?

SUMMARY OF HEALTHCARE PROFESSIONALS AND THEIR SKILLS IN PAIN MANAGEMENT

Healthcare professional	Skills + management they offer	Support self-management skills in these areas
General practitioner/ family physician	Assesses and diagnoses types of pain, including acute and chronic. Prescribes trials of medication to lessen pain and reviews and reduces where medicines are harmful or unhelpful, e.g. strong opioids. Investigates and makes specialist service referral for further assessment and management. Diagnoses other conditions that add to the impact of pain, such as depression, other health problems like diabetes and sleep disorders. Treats these conditions or refer to specialist services.	Enables the person to know about the difference between acute and chronic pain. Advises on ways to use and stop medicines safely. Encourages setting of personal goals, improving fitness, healthy eating and lifestyle and balancing activities. Supports and helps modify setback plans. Advises on trusted sources of coaching and support for self-management within the local community.
Practice nurse/ nurse practitioner	Assessment, and identification with the person, of their needs due to pain and priorities. Helps with making plans on ways to self-manage pain and maintain health. Identifies any life or mood issues that need more help and assessment. Shares healthy living activities and services in the community to build fitness, relaxation, etc.	Enables the person to know about the difference between acute and chronic pain. Encourages setting of personal goals, improving fitness, healthy eating and lifestyle and balancing activities. Supports and helps modify setback plans. Advises on trusted sources of coaching and support for self-management within the local community.

Healthcare professional	Skills + management they offer	Support self-management skills in these areas
Physiotherapist	Understands how to assess the impact of pain on the individual. Assesses body movements and physical activities. Plans with the person ways to reduce disability through individual specific physical movement programmes. Has awareness of mood issues and pain, especially fears about movement and pain.	Knowledge of pain, brain and nervous system. Balancing daily activities (pacing). How to set a range of goals. Building fitness, improving balance. Using and choosing relaxation options. Managing setbacks/maintaining progress. Helping with acceptance that pain is long term. Advises on sleeping well.
Pain medicine specialist	Diagnoses types of chronic pain conditions. Assesses the impact of pain on the individual. Manages a range of medications and other interventions to reduce some pain symptoms. Refers to other health teams to address practical ways to manage pain, moods, fitness, work issues, relationships, etc.	Guides safe use of medicines. Guides safe use of pain treatment devices.

Specialist pain management nurse	Knows about pain, brain and nerve network function. Supports use of a range of medications and other treatments. Identifies severe mood changes for further assessment.	Assessing and guiding safe use of medicines and treatment devices. Monitoring change/progress of pain experience. Similar to the physiotherapist in supporting skills in pacing activities, setting range of goals, developing setback plans, better sleep skills.
Talking therapist	Understands the emotions, thinking and behaviours linked to pain.	Helps you learn and use the Five-Areas CBT tool. Guides you through it to develop your own management of pain. Helps build a range of skills from pacing, goal setting and sleeping well. Supports ways to manage moods and unhelpful thinking patterns. Helps develop patterns of kindness and to reduce negative and critical assessment of self. Guides setback planning.

These healthcare professionals also help the people around you, like your family and carers. They can guide them concerning ways to support you positively that build your confidence to manage your pain well. They can offer helpful guidance and support to other clinicians as well.

Sometimes you can benefit from the support of other professionals, such as counsellors, fitness instructors, health coaches, art therapists or social workers.

What are the roles of healthcare professionals?

The roles of the general practitioner/family physician and primary care nurse/nurse practitioner

These professionals are most likely to look after your day-to-day healthcare issues in the long term. More about their roles are shared in the table above. They can support you directly to gain more skills and tools to manage pain. They often have a lot of knowledge of local services, so may refer you to the physiotherapy team for pain management or other pain specialist services.

They can link you to resources like trusted books, web-based resources and community support, local self-help groups; they also know of specific services or courses that would fit your needs. Sometimes specialist services are very useful: when or if your confidence to cope with pain is very low; or when you are experiencing a lot of mood issues such as depression; or when pain is proving very limiting physically, as in Mo's story; or when there are harmful problems linked to medication.

In Chapter 1 you may have looked at how pain was controlling you and your life →: page 6. If your score was eight or more out of ten, share this with your family doctor, together with your score on your confidence level to make changes →: page 25. If your confidence level is low – less than three – and the pain controlling your life is eight or more, then discuss with your GP/family doctor or nurse about referral to specialist pain management services.

The role of the physiotherapist (physical therapist)

Physiotherapists have specialist knowledge, skills and experience of the musculoskeletal system and the pain system, and understand how the nerves, bones, muscles and tendons, joints and ligaments work together. They assess how your body moves and functions and then work with you to change or improve your physical abilities and health.

Physiotherapists understand the way the body works in lots of day-to-day situations, like:

- walking on the flat or uneven surfaces;
- going up and down stairs;
- bending down to pick something up or reaching up to a shelf;
- putting your socks on, brushing your hair;

- getting in and out of a bath or shower, chair, car or bus;
- riding a bike, swimming or walking;
- playing sports, e.g. ball games or tennis, golf.

Some physiotherapists specialise in pain management. They have extra training in building confidence and managing pain better, as in Mo's example. They will work with people either one to one or in small groups. Sometimes they have extra training in talking therapies, such as using cognitive behavioural therapy approaches (CBT), and some may be able to prescribe medicines, although most physiotherapists do not prescribe.

A **pain management physiotherapist** supports you to build your skills and resources, by helping you to:

- create a specific personal exercise programme to build stamina, strength and flexibility.
- pace your daily activities.
- find helpful sleep positions and sleep well skills.
- set goals in order to achieve things.
- solve problems and adapt to any physical limitations you might have.
- increase your physical fitness with no, or minimal, change in your pain.
- manage setbacks.
- use relaxation skills to manage yourself and your pain better.
- address fears about movements and pain.

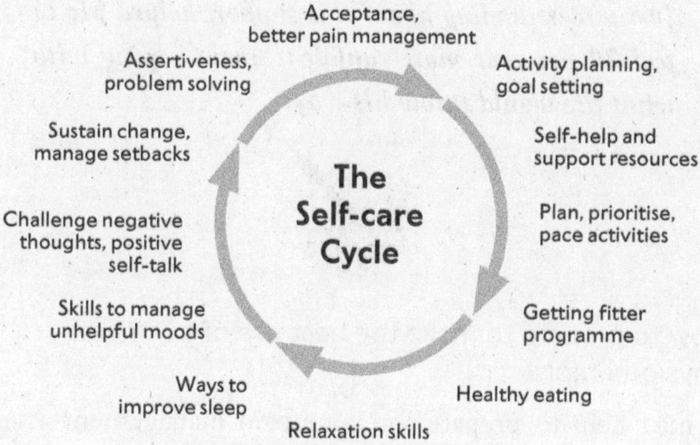

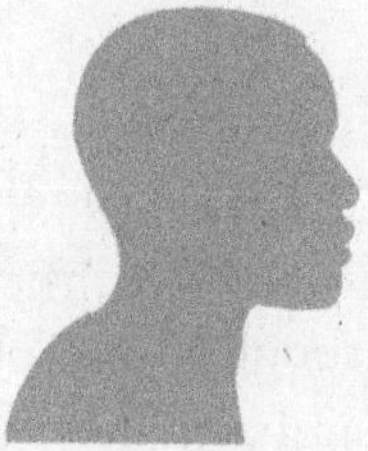

Mo realised that he needed help using the stairs. He avoided the home stairs as much as possible as he had slipped on them twice, which made his pain much worse. He was now frightened to use the stairs and climbing down them made him panic.

He and his physiotherapist made a plan to help Mo with the use of stairs and in other ways. These included pacing his activities, improving his sleeping positions and stretching and strengthening muscles so that he could stand and walk for longer.

Just understanding about this support helped Mo to feel 20 per cent more confident about coping with what life would throw his way.

How to prepare to make the best use of a physiotherapist

It may help to prepare for your pain management assessment with a specialist physiotherapist or any healthcare professional by trying one or more of these three actions:

- Check out the pain cycle and tick off your three priority areas for change now →: page 28.
- Making notes about how your pain affects your day-to-day physical activities and other areas such as moods.
- Write down any questions to ask them about pain and self-management.

The role of the specialist pain management nurse

These nurses have specialist training in working with patients with chronic pain, and with their families. They usually work with pain medicine specialist doctors in hospitals, sometimes in the community and often with members of specialist pain management teams.

A **specialist pain management nurse** helps you to:

- Use pain-relief medicines safely to reduce their harmful short- and long-term side-effects.
- Find better timings to fit the taking of medicines into your day and night routines.
- Reduce medicines safely, especially strong opioids and gabapentinoids.
- Track what difference pain-relief medicines make to your ability to achieve your own goals and action plans.
- Support your efforts to use non-drug approaches to manage pain, especially during setbacks.
- Link you to other sources of support within the pain management service or other services that can help you to live well.

The role of a pain medicine specialist

Pain medicine specialists are medically trained and trained in anaesthetics, an area of medical care that enables people to have pain-free operations. As Jim explained to Anne his wife, 'They put you to sleep before an operation.' These doctors have a range of skills in different pain-reducing treatments and they are skilled in reducing pain in acute or cancer-related pain cases. Their role in chronic pain is different.

When a pain medicine specialist supports someone with chronic pain, they usually carry out a person-centred assessment of the pain problem. These specialists may suggest a trial of different medicines for a set period, usually eight to twelve weeks, or offer a trial of a course of injections or similar treatments of pain-reducing medicines around the nerves near the pain areas. These may reduce *some* pain for certain periods of time – perhaps a few weeks.

The focus of the treatments is to make it easier to start personal goals, make helpful changes to daily activities and build confidence in your own self-management. It is tricky though, as sometimes they can make pain symptoms worse or make no difference, leaving a sense of failure and frustration. These medicines or other options are not seen by specialists as a long-term treatment. They are stopped after such a trial if they fail to help the person to self-manage confidently, as they can cause harmful side-effects. For example, if the person fails to achieve set personal goals or if emotional and physical health have not improved or worsened.

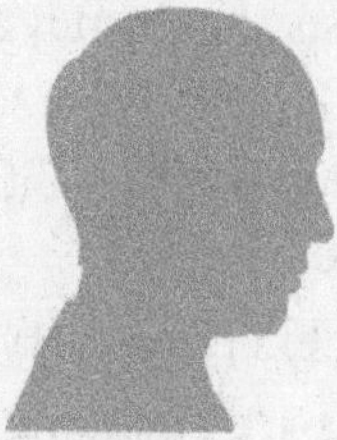

Jim realised that a pain-relieving injection had once helped Anne's shoulder. He asked the physiotherapist, 'Would something like this help me?' Lee, the physiotherapist, explained that 'it was pot luck that they help in chronic pain. Anne had an acute pain problem with her shoulder. An injection treatment is helpful in this specific shoulder problem as it is acute, not chronic.'

Jim asked the pain medicine specialist, too. She shared that injections are used in some pain conditions and usually done as a trial of injections over several weeks. They can have side-effects and sometimes even make the pain worse. 'Pain is complicated' and 'in your case we should support your self-management goals and action plans to manage the pain. This will be more helpful and safer long term.'

After talking with Anne, Jim decided he would concentrate his efforts on the personal exercise and relaxation programme he was learning with the support of the physiotherapist. He realised that looking for solutions for his pain through injections sadly was not realistic.

Pain medicine specialists sometimes carry out investigations to see if there are any specific causes of chronic pain. This can then make it easier to plan different ways to reduce some of the pain levels.

A specialist is more likely to carry out tests or investigations if your symptoms are changing or if they are unusual, such as numbness, loss of feeling in the arms or legs, loss of bladder or bowel control, or great difficulty in walking.

The role of specialist psychologists and CBT talking therapists

Psychologists and CBT psychotherapists have specific training to understand the way a person thinks and feels about themselves, their pain, the world around them and other people. As you will have seen in Chapter 1, the Five-Areas tool is a CBT model used for managing your pain, and psychologists and talking therapists will use this model to guide therapy.

Their role is to work with people to understand the way a person's mind and body work together with their health or pain problem. This enables them to guide a person with chronic pain to understand how and why the pain affects their moods, thoughts and behaviours, their current life situation and other people. They are trained in working with people who have anxiety, depression and other mental health problems, as well as specifically living with pain ➔: page 237.

FIVE AREAS

- Body symptoms, such as pain, tiredness, sleep, etc.
- Thoughts, memories, images and beliefs about the pain.
- Moods or emotions.
- Actions or behaviours.
- What is currently happening in your life situation or happened in the past.

A **specialist psychologist or CBT psychotherapist (talking therapist)** can help you to:

- Understand your reactions to upsetting or traumatic experiences in your life, like serious illness or family problems.
- Manage or cope better with distressing mental health symptoms such as depression, anxiety, panic attacks, anger, eating disorders and Obsessive Compulsive Disorder.
- Understand that mental health problems are common – one in four people have mental health problems at some point in their lives.
- Cope with the emotional upset and distress of living with a long-term physical illness like chronic pain.

- Cope with your reactions to losses that you have experienced due to pain, such as loss of work or independence.
- Help you to be compassionate to yourself, by being kinder, supportive, less judgemental and less self-critical.

As part of the pain management team, psychologists and CBT therapists work with other healthcare practitioners such as pain medicine specialists or psychiatrists or rehabilitation professionals like physiotherapists. They may be a doctor of psychology, but they do not prescribe medicines.

They may work one to one with an individual and may also support family members. They can bring together, in groups, patients who share common problems, to work with them on areas like anxiety, worry or pain, using Cognitive Behavioural Therapy or other therapy options. See more on pain management programmes below →: page 105.

In some situations, you can refer yourself to a psychologist or psychotherapist for help with mental health issues and management of long-term physical conditions. You may also be referred by your GP or hospital specialist.

Why work with a psychologist or CBT psychotherapist?

If you are struggling to self-manage sleeping, your mood, or feel that anxiety, frustration or worry is getting too much, this may be the time to seek extra help. If you are finding it difficult to see people; or your loved ones are concerned about you, that is a good reason to speak to someone who can work with you to overcome this.

Seeing someone who is trained in psychology or talking therapies does not mean that your pain is 'all in your mind'. Other people around you may say this to you, which is **totally unhelpful**; it shows they do not understand. We now know that all pain is actually processed within the brain and so it makes better sense to work with both 'mind' and body.

What happens when I see a talking therapist?

Normally you will be invited to a one-to-one assessment session and the therapist will work with you to understand more about yourself and how your pain is affecting you as a person, including your thinking, feelings and what you do. They are likely to ask about the impact on relationships with others, and how you cope with the pain at the moment.

In CBT, for example, they may focus on the 'Five Areas' at first, →: page 9, and draw out how these all interact with each other.

The next step is to understand:

- What aspects of your moods, thinking and behaviours might be improved through different talking therapy approaches.
- What things can be changed to help you to manage your pain, and live well.
- How you can work together to make a plan to reach your goals. This might mean trying out new things or changing the way you approach what you are doing already.
- Ways to challenge unhelpful thoughts, or manage activity levels by pacing.
- Ways of coming to terms with the losses you experience and reaching a place of acceptance.

The overall focus is to help you find and use many strategies to increase confidence in managing and living well with pain.

The role of talking therapies

Chronic pain can be a distressing and miserable experience, making you feel quite alone and different from other people.

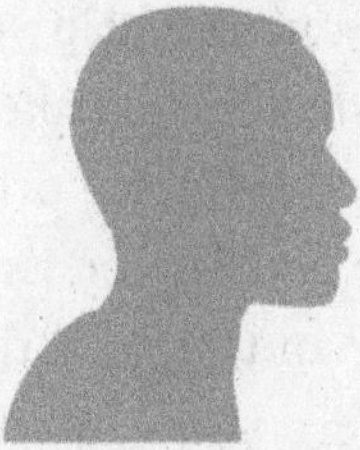

Mo certainly felt that his parents and friends couldn't understand what he was going through, which made him feel worse. His accident left him with lots of fears. He went for some CBT talking therapy sessions and this helped him to share the ways in which the pain had changed his thinking patterns, and affected his mood and activity levels. Mo used his talking therapy sessions to tackle these things, including his fear of falling and why he avoided the use of stairs. This meant he had lost his fitness and felt unsteady when walking. He saw himself getting weaker and feeble, so he felt depressed →: page 290. *He lost confidence in his ability to tackle the stairs; it was like a vicious cycle of doom!*

CBT talking therapy was able to help Mo:

- *to tackle his fear of using the stairs, which, in turn, benefited his fitness and moods;*
- *to discover more about how to change his thinking about life situations, pain and other people, so he became less anxious and stressed;*
- *to agree that a pain management programme might be a useful choice* →: overleaf.

CBT talking therapies can also help you to explore past life events that may overshadow or take hold of your mind, leaving you feeling angry, worried or depressed. It can help you to deal with sleep and fatigue issues by changing how you manage both day and night activities. CBT can help you reach a place where you can accept the changes that have happened because of your pain, including losses. It can help to increase your awareness of positive or useful aspects of change.

Research has shown that CBT can be helpful in treating many different mental health problems, including depression, anxiety, panic attacks and post-traumatic stress disorder. CBT can also be used to help manage physical health problems, such as chronic pain, and other chronic illnesses, such as heart failure and sleep problems.

What is the role of a psychiatrist in pain management?

Psychiatrists are medical doctors who specialise in mental illness such as severe depression, anxiety or other mental health problems, such as schizophrenia.

In chronic pain, where there can be complex problems, psychiatrists assess or diagnose a person's mental health difficulties and suggest talking or other therapies or drug treatments. They may prescribe a trial of medicines, for example, to reduce levels of anxiety or depression and review progress in benefit from them and any side-effects or harm.

Some psychiatrists have expertise in managing addiction problems too, which is useful as sometimes people can become dependent on strong pain medicines such as opioids (including morphine) or certain medicines used to manage nerve or neuropathic pain.

Psychiatrists work within a team of mental health professionals and will refer to the team for help, using talking therapies or additional support in teaching practical skills to manage mental health problems.

Other sources of pain management support

What are pain management programmes?

These programmes are for groups of people with a range of pain issues, led by healthcare professionals. They help people learn self-management skills to cope with life better, despite the pain persisting.

Meeting every week for a few weeks, the programme will involve learning about pain, and practising new skills to manage it better. Being in a group means that people can learn from each other and support each other.

It's a bit like going on a part-time course to learn to manage your pain better and you then get to try out your new skills at home. Many people with chronic pain have found these programmes very helpful.

What sort of pain management programme (PMP) might be valuable?

There is a range of options and it depends on what extent the pain impacts on you and your health and confidence levels. Some programmes are run in specialist pain management centres, others are run in the community by specialist pain management teams or by a range of self-help groups or health charities. If pain has a big impact on all areas of your Five-Areas tool and your confidence to cope is less than three out of ten, then a specialist PMP service is likely to be best. Pain self-management-skills group-based community programmes are usually suitable for people where pain is affecting them in certain areas and their confidence-to-cope levels are between four to seven out of ten.

What do PMPs focus on to help with self-management?

They help people to know more about:

- pain and the brain systems, and how pain works; →: page 52.
- medicines and ways to manage them safely; →: page 377.

To develop confidence to learn and grow skills in:

- getting fitter and more active, and using stretching and strengthening exercises to regain or increase fitness; →: page 150.
- using pacing of activities to help reduce severe pain levels; →: page 125.
- setting goals for relaxation, social and enjoyable activities; →: page 174.
- solving problems; →: page 327.
- rewarding yourself; →: page 112.

- maintaining positive changes using fitness and pacing activities.
- ways to sleep well.
- talking through difficulties with others, especially partners and family; →: page 212.
- managing moods, such as depression, anger and worry, or anxiety →: page 290 and the impact of loss.
- using relaxation skills, such as deep breathing, or relaxing imagery or sounds, or meditation; →: page 174.
- coping well with setbacks and planning for positive future journeys →: page 319.
- ways to support each other positively and deal with loss and changes.

A person who attended a pain management programme shared with Mo:

> *I was able to move forward and learn to cope and accept my pain. The group support from others, who knew what it was like to deal with the pain, made a big difference. They really understood and offered different ways and ideas to deal with problems. It helped my family, as they realised that more activities were possible if I paced myself better. My frustration lessened and I was able to laugh again.*

After a pain management programme, you can expect to (tick any of the points below you would choose to do):

- Return to or take up new activities, hobbies, to visit friends and family, etc.
- Do more enjoyable and rewarding activities with family, friends.
- Return to work, often through special schemes that may be available locally.
- Develop confidence in the ability to . . .
  1. Communicate your needs better to your family, work or colleagues, or your doctor.
  2. Manage setbacks a little better.
  3. Improve your ability to tackle and solve problems.
  4. Develop your skills such as pacing, goal setting and relaxation.
- Start a study or computer course.
- Start voluntary work or a new role for a few hours each week.
- Get involved with art, crafts or music.

Chapter summary

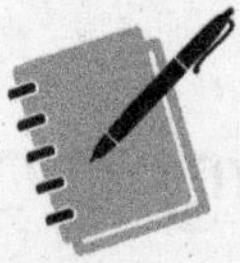

- A range of different healthcare professionals can be an invaluable guide to support you to manage pain better, and its effects on moods and thinking, physical activity and life, despite the pain.
- It helps to work with your GP/family doctor/nurse to discover what self-management support and service could be useful to build your confidence.
- Talking therapies can offer a chance to talk through life changes resulting from pain, as well as ways of coping with pain and its effects on moods, thoughts, actions and your life situation.
- Pain management programmes are a useful way to learn more about chronic pain and how to cope with it better.
- To help you gain these skills, these programmes involve working with a group of people who also struggle with pain. Support is provided by other pain sufferers in the group and by healthcare staff.

5

Reaching goals and creating rewards

What this chapter covers

In this chapter we will take a look at goals and rewards. Goals are a helpful way of noticing and recording the progress you make over time. Sometimes, for people with chronic pain, goals may take longer to achieve and require more planning to begin with. However, this doesn't mean they are impossible. Goal setting helps you get back control in many different areas of your life; for example, hobbies, work, taking less medication and developing a better sleep pattern.

Rewards are tiny treats or pleasures that can provide a boost when you are working towards goals. They could be things like a trip to the movies, spending some time in the garden, or having afternoon tea with a friend.

How goals and rewards help with managing chronic pain

Goals can help you focus on what's important or of value to you. They help you make progress and this, in turn, will increase your self-confidence. Goals help you to focus on the things that matter most to you. You can set goals related to any area of your life; think about the person-centred Five-Areas tool →: page 9. For example, you might want to be more physically active, so you could set yourself a goal to swim twelve lengths of the local pool twice a week, to be achieved over a three-month period. Or you may want to socialise more, in which case you might set a goal of having a family meal out, going and listening to a band, or a half-day shopping trip to the mall with friends, once a month.

Rewards give a sense of pleasure, satisfaction or achievement and help build confidence. They give us the drive to try something new, even when it seems difficult. They encourage us to think 'it's worth a try'. Rewards help us to repeat activities, especially when learning new skills. We tend to do more of something if we feel rewarded for it, either by ourselves or by others.

Useful things to know about goals and goal setting

Goals are things that you wish to achieve, either for yourself or with others, despite having chronic pain. It can be helpful to think of your goals as if they are an end destination. If the destination is close, then goals will be short term.

Alternatively, if your sights are set far in the distance, then it may be long-term goals that you need.

When you set goals, you need to think about how you will achieve them. What kind of journey are you going to take? For people who live with chronic pain, setting goals and working towards them can be a challenge. Rather like a train taking you on a journey, they may have to take detours, deal with delays, faults on the line or timetable changes; but in the end, they will get there. People who live with pain tell us that goal setting is a very useful skill that helps them to live a better life, despite the pain.

Rewards give a sense of pleasure or achievement. An ice cream can be a reward; so can a pay packet at the end of the week; a game of cards with a friend; a clean kitchen floor; or a 'well done' note to yourself. Rewards vary according to the individual. Something that is a reward for one person may not be seen as a reward by another.

Learning the skills to set goals

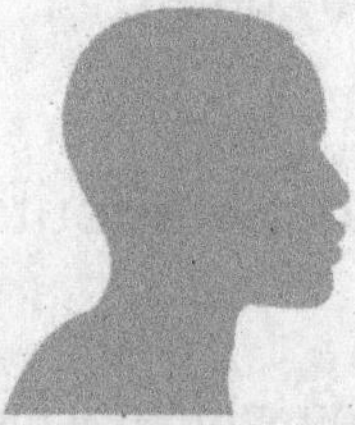

Let's start by taking a look at Mo. *He has some difficulties around his sleep pattern. Due to pain, he stays up very late and then sleeps in until the afternoon. He tells*

his parents, 'I am not coming downstairs, I'm staying in my room. It's close to the toilet and my computer is there.' Some days he stays in his bedroom almost all day, spending most of his time either sat down at his computer or lying on his bed. He finds his dad's walking stick helpful, but refuses to go outside with it in case someone sees him. He has tried at least six or seven different types of pain medication, but he finds that they only work for the first two or three weeks. He is not keen to try any more and is fed-up with their side-effects, especially constipation and a dry mouth. He is no longer able to continue his hobbies or work. Mo often thinks about all the things he used to do, such as cycling on Saturdays and canoeing with his friends.

These are the kinds of difficulties that Mo is likely to have with goal setting:

- *He can't imagine how things could be different – he feels trapped in the situation he is in.*
- *He wouldn't know where to start, as there are so many things in his life that he is unhappy with.*
- *He is worried that if he tries to do more, he will make his pain worse.*
- *He is too tired and lacking in energy to think about changing anything.*
- *The side-effects of his medicines mean that his head is too fuzzy to think about anything for long.*
- *He prefers not to think about his hobbies and interests, as it just reminds him of what he has lost as a result of his accident.*

What thoughts and feelings do you have about goal setting? Use the space below to list any of the obstacles that might get in the way of setting and achieving your goals.

____

____

____

____

____

____

____

____

How **confident** are you in goal setting?

0 1 2 3 4 5 6 7 8 9 10

Not at all confident — Extremely confident

How **confident** are you in achieving your goals?

0 1 2 3 4 5 6 7 8 9 10

Not at all confident — Extremely confident

Mo is able to identify three goals:

1. Be able to go outside without the need for a walking stick.
2. Get back to cycling.
3. Slowly stop taking all pain medicines.

This is a good start, but these goals are still a bit vague, so with the help of his parents he was able to make them SMART. This involved making sure that each of his goals are:

Specific – states exactly what will be achieved.

Measurable – says how often something will happen and for how long.

Achievable – is realistic.

Rewarding – is enjoyable.

Timed – states how much time is needed to achieve a goal.

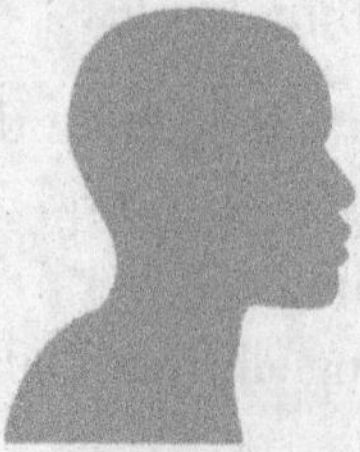

Mo's SMART goals looked like this:
By the end of this month I will . . .

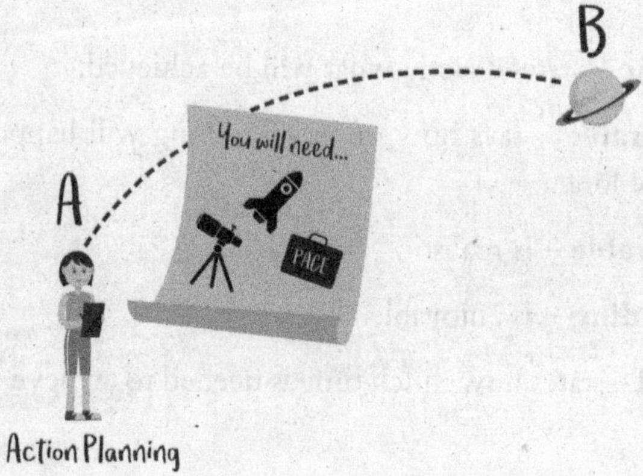

1. *Go to the shops and back without using the walking stick at least three times a week.*
2. *Get my bike out of the shed and give it the 'once-over' and check the brakes and tyres.*
3. *Talk to my GP about how to phase out my pain medicines and get a plan in place to do this.*

SMART goal setting is a skill that will give you a clear view of what you want to achieve in a set timeframe. It will help you plan how you get there and continue to reach goals successfully. Sharing your goals with other people helps them to understand what matters to you and how they can help you make progress. All these factors will increase your chances of success, and you can start planning the reward/s now!

Remember to evaluate or assess and, if necessary, revise your goals as you go along. Making a goal SMART means your goals should provide:

- a bit of a challenge *and* not be so difficult that you find that your pain or stiffness become more difficult to manage;
- the ability to revise or adjust them if problems emerge with pain, setbacks or life issues.

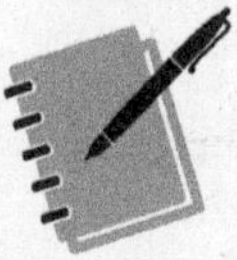

Have a look at the table below and choose at least two areas where you would like to set yourself a goal.

Have a go at writing a SMART goal for each area that you choose.

Use the examples to give yourself ideas, e.g. Razia's goal planning steps ➔: page 120.

Area of my life	For example, this could be . . .	My SMART goals (no need to fill in all areas)
Social/fun activities	Go out for a meal, watch a film, have a coffee with a friend, do craftwork, plant up a flowerbed.	
Work	Paid or voluntary, staying in current role, reduce/increase hours, retrain.	
Hobbies	Gardening, fishing, drama, walking, guitar.	
Household tasks	Changing and making beds, cooking meals, vacuuming, cleaning, managing finances.	
Physical activity	Stretches, football in park, yoga, swimming.	
Caring for myself	Having a bath, putting my own socks and shoes on, cooking a nice meal.	

Tools and resources that can support you to make changes →: page 349.

Okay, now you've set some SMART goals, how do you make sure that you achieve them?

Sometimes it's worth thinking about your SMART goals like steps on a ladder. This will help you to break each goal down into smaller achievable steps, week by week, to build up to the bigger goal. You could estimate each step may take about a week to achieve. Razia's example below may help you plan the steps and ways to deal with difficulties.

For each of your weekly steps, think about the things that will help your progress and those that could block you. This will help you to work out what you need to do to increase your chance of success.

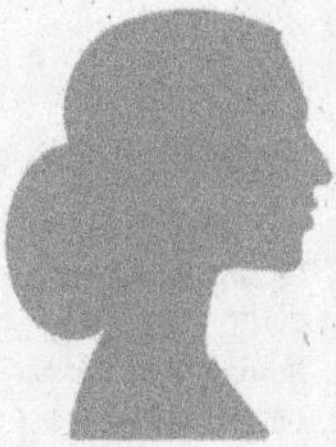

Razia wanted to cook a family meal. It was to be part of a special meal celebration for her friends and family. She wanted to cook both a main course and a dessert. The meal itself is in three weeks' time.

This she made into a SMART goal, which was:

- *To cook two courses of a family meal for a celebration in three weeks' time.*

This is what she told us she planned and did.

Razia's SMART Goal Steps to Make Dinner For Friends and Family

	Activities to help me achieve my goal	Things that will help my progress	Things that might block my progress
Week 3	Make dessert on Saturday morning. Ask Hassan to prepare carrots and potatoes on Sunday.	My eldest son wants to help make the dessert, too.	Table will be too small – I need to work out how I can make it bigger.
Week 2	Write list of foods to make so I can pace myself. Check dessert recipe. Make shopping list and buy food needed. Try out dessert recipe on the family on Friday night.	Plan ahead with a reward: watch my favourite wildlife film. Borrow Mum's easy recipe book as the family loved the dessert last time.	My youngest son is not very well – so less time to prepare.
Start Week 1	Find out what cooking equipment I need. Make a list of what I need to use or do. Arrange to have the oven fixed. Find the hand mixer. Check if any foods are unsuitable or disliked.	Use a recipe that I know well. Contact people by text early evening.	Oven isn't working well. Can't find my mixer – need to get family to look for it.

My goal: *'Make dinner for friends and family in three weeks' time.'*

Now have a go at writing your week-by-week steps for your own goals, using the blank goal ladder overleaf, and involve others if that helps →: page 122.

- Ask yourself what goal would make an immediate positive change.
- Write down one goal, then fill in the steps on the goal ladder for the first week.

If it seems a struggle, try a fun or rewarding goal. Avoid a chore or really tricky goal, like losing weight, as these can demotivate you.

Sometimes, to get started, experiment and try an easy goal. People with pain often aim too high, or to do things too early or quickly, and this pattern of 'overachieving' often leads to repeated setbacks.

Remember to build in regular rewards for yourself along the way.

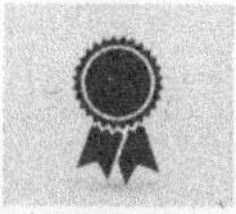

My SMART goal at the end of __________ weeks

is to ______________________________________

My Goal Ladder

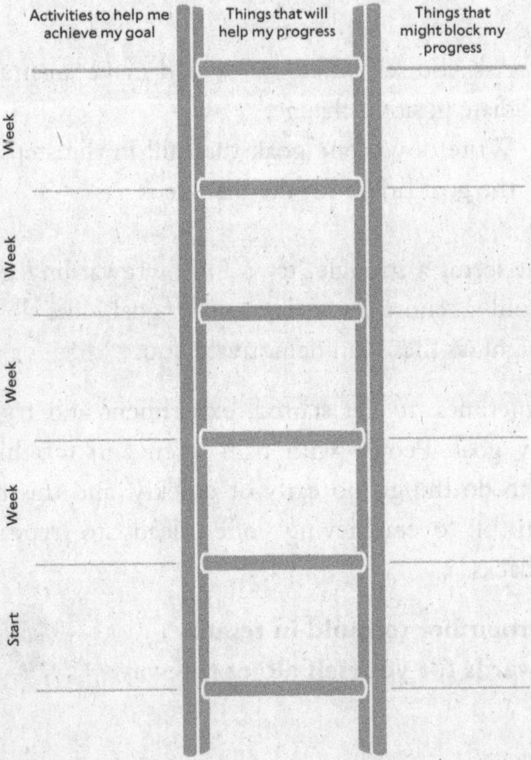

What do you plan as a reward for your efforts and your achievement?

____

____

Self-check on progress

As you go forward and set goals for the future, you may want to:

- Continue to build on the same goals, for example, doing something for longer, with people, in a different place, and so on.
- Maintain the same goals.
- Choose different goals in other areas (see the table →: page 118 for ideas) or experiment with new activities.

Dealing with setbacks

Remember, sometimes things happen that get in the way of achieving your goals. This could include illness, lack of money, or appointments at the hospital. Try not to lose hope or confidence when this happens. You can stay on the same step of the ladder for a week or more, until you are ready to move on. Explore the chapter on setbacks for more information →: page 319.

Chapter summary

- Goal setting is a valuable skill to help make positive changes in the different areas of your life.
- With SMART planning, goal setting can be an enjoyable, rewarding experience. Remember that it takes time to become confident in regularly using this skill.
- Rewarding successes or progress in small steps on the goal ladder helps to keep motivation going and build self-confidence.

6

Balancing daily activities through pacing

What this chapter covers

People living with chronic pain find that pacing is one of the key everyday skills to learn and use. In this chapter you will find out what pacing means and discover the benefits of balancing activities through the day. We will share resources that will help you to plan your activities and breaks. This is so that you can achieve your goals without increasing your pain or letting tiredness force you to stop. You'll find how pacing is like the story of the tortoise and hare: slow and steady wins the race.

What is the value of pacing in managing chronic pain?

Healthcare professionals and people living with pain use the term pacing, describing it as 'an active self-management skill where the individual balances time spent on activity and rest for the overall purpose of achieving a gradual increase in the range of tasks, activities and roles over time'. Put another way, it is about choosing when to take a break from an activity without being forced to stop by pain, tiredness or other symptoms, not '*letting pain be your guide*' or a trigger to stop and rest.

Here are some of the positive changes that people with pain noticed after they learnt the skills of pacing and balancing their range of activities.

DOING MORE: They could do more over time, either by themselves or with family and friends. They could tick more things off their 'to-do' list.

SLEEPING BETTER: They could sleep better at night.

MORE CONTROL: They felt they had more control over the pain and their activity levels.

LESS MEDICATION: They depended less on medications and thus experienced fewer unpleasant side-effects.

BRIGHTER MOODS: Life became more enjoyable – they had more fun.

MORE ENERGY: They felt stronger and more energetic – they had more 'get up and go'.

A BETTER SOCIAL LIFE: With more confidence that their pain was manageable, they could plan for a better social life and do more things with family and friends.

LESS PAIN: They found they had less pain and had fewer setbacks, which didn't last long.

LESS EFFORT: They felt less effort was required to achieve daily tasks and activities.

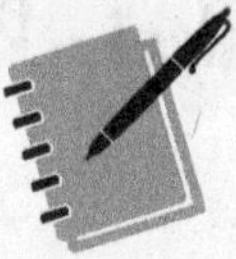

Explore the above benefits of pacing that people with pain have noticed.

Which two or three of these benefits most appeal to you?

____

____

____

Useful things to know about unhelpful pacing

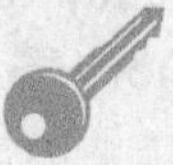

Generally, there are two styles of pacing for people with chronic pain: overactive, underactive. Both styles have advantages and disadvantages. As you read about the pacing styles below, decide which pacing style you currently use; it may be a mixture of both.

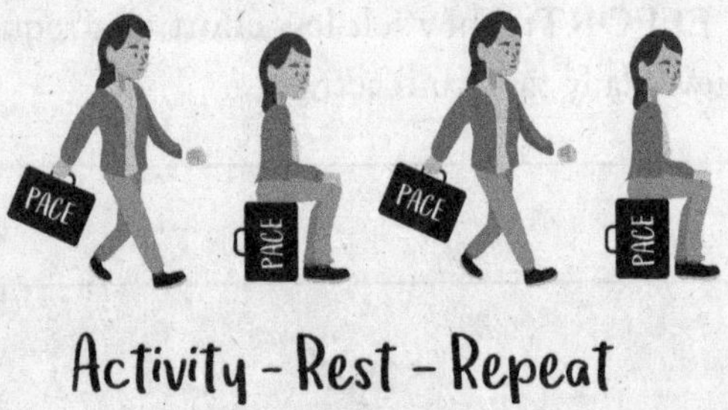

Overactive pacing

This means doing too much activity or too many tasks over a short space of time. It may happen if you are having a good day, with less pain, or your mood is better →: page 237. This sounds a little like Jim's style of pacing. He is trying to do too much and ends up with more pain and tiredness. This means he misses out on enjoyable things like gardening.

Underactive pacing

This means that you are doing too little activity to help keep strength, stamina and flexibility in your muscles, ligaments, joints and bones. More of your time is spent resting, sitting or lying down, which is understandable, especially if there is a lot of pain. However, it may in turn add to your pain, as lack of fitness makes muscles and other tissues tight, weak and painful. Mo's current pacing style looks underactive, and he appears to be doing less and less because of the pain and his fear of going up and down stairs → : page 6.

Mixed pacing style

Very often people with pain use pain and energy levels as a guide to their activities and pacing them. This means they risk doing too much activity on good days, which then makes their pain worse. They are forced to rest while the pain settles down, sometimes for a couple of days. This is a **mixed style** of pacing, which is unhelpful in the long term, sometimes known as 'boom and bust'.

Let's explore the issues that Jim and Mo have with pacing.

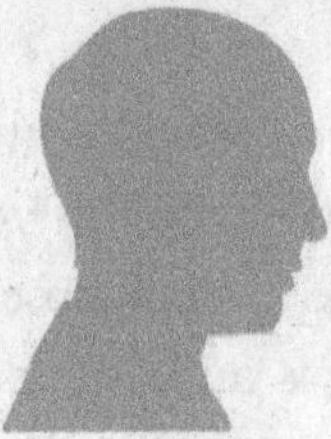

Jim keeps himself very busy most days doing household chores, such as vacuuming, shopping, cooking and cleaning; he keeps going by telling himself, 'It helps to keep busy as it takes my mind off the pain.' However, he has noticed that there is no time any more to do the things he enjoys, like gardening. He says, 'I am tired, my pain feels worse, I am stuck in a vicious cycle.' Jim tries to do everything at once and only stops when he is forced to, due to increases in pain and tiredness.

Do you recognise yourself in Jim's story? What would you advise him to do to balance his activities?

Jim's story is a common experience for many people with chronic pain – it is an **overactive style of activity**.

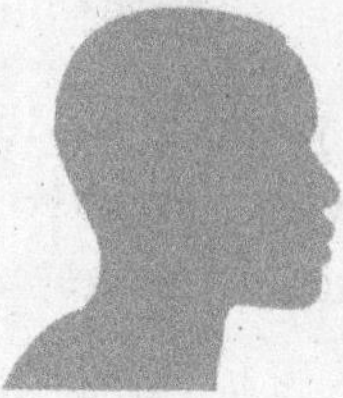

Let's consider Mo's experience. He spends much of his time sleeping, sitting or lying down to try to manage his pain. He has limited his physical activity as he believes this will control his pain and symptoms. However, he has noticed that the pain doesn't get easier if he rests more and he is achieving less on a day-to-day basis. He is losing the fitness and flexibility he used to have. He tries to do more on good days, but then 'pays for it' later when pain and muscle soreness get the better of him. When this happens, he is forced to go to bed for several hours to rest.

Mo's story is a common experience for many people with chronic pain who use their level of pain to guide the amount of activity they do on a daily basis. Mo does more on good days, then is forced to rest. This style of activity is called a ***'boom and bust' cycle****.*

Do you recognise yourself in Mo's story? If Mo was your best friend, what would you suggest to him to do to manage his daily activity?

Understanding more about your pacing style

In order to learn how to pace well, it's important to understand what your pacing style is now. A good way to do this is to track your activities with a daily diary like the one below. Let's take a look at Jim and what he did on Wednesday morning.

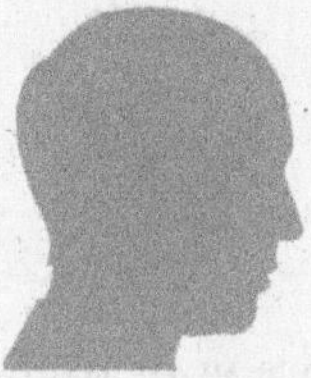

JIM'S DAILY DIARY: MY TYPICAL DAY

Time	Day, e.g. Wednesday	How many minutes did you do?
6 a.m.	Sleep	
7 a.m.	Sleep	
8 a.m.	Shower. Got dressed. Made me and Anne some breakfast.	10 5 20
9 a.m.	Washed the dishes and tidied the kitchen. Put some washing into the machine.	25 5
10 a.m.	Sat with Anne and had a coffee and a chat. Looked through the kitchen cupboards and wrote the shopping list for today's groceries.	30 10
11 a.m.	Changed the sheets on our bed and vacuumed upstairs. Hung out the washing for it to dry. Sat and read the daily newspaper.	30 15 15
12 p.m.	Got ready to leave the house and go shopping. Collected the shopping bags; hunted for the car keys, as they were lost. Got into the car and drove to the supermarket.	10 5 20

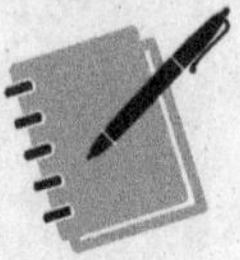

Now start to explore your pacing style.
Fill in the Pacing Diary below for at least two days.
To do this you will need to:

- shade in the boxes for the hours when you were asleep;
- write what you were doing and for how many minutes each time;
- write down when you took a break, sat down or lay down, and for how long.

PACING DIARY: MY TYPICAL DAY

Time	Day, e.g. Wednesday	How many minutes did you do?
6 a.m.		
7 a.m.		
8 a.m.		
9 a.m.		
10 a.m.		
11 a.m.		

12 p.m.		
1 p.m.		
2 p.m.		
3 p.m.		
4 p.m.		
5 p.m.		
6 p.m.		
7 p.m.		
8 p.m.		
9 p.m.		
10 p.m.		
11 p.m.		
12 a.m.		
1 a.m.		
2 a.m.		
3 a.m.		
4 a.m.		
5 a.m.		

When you have completed your Pacing Diary, what do you notice about your pacing style? Use our questions to guide your thinking.

REVIEW YOUR PACING DIARY

Have a look at what you have written in your diary and answer these questions:

How much activity did you do each day?
__________________ hours or minutes

How much time did you spend resting, sitting or lying down each day?
__________________ hours or minutes

How many hours were you asleep each day?
__________________ hours or minutes

Did you manage to do the things you needed to do? If yes which ones?

____

How much effort did your activities take on a scale of 0________________10 (see scale on page 138)?

Do you think your current pacing style is mainly **underactive**, like Mo's, or **overactive**, like Jim's, or a **mixture** of both styles?

____

Tools and resources that can help you to pace well

There are different ways to make some changes to your pacing style. Here are some suggestions and ways to experiment.

Effort levels – a further useful way to pace well

Check the effort levels of the activity and use the skill of matching effort levels and activity to make certain the balance is right for the situation or plan.

A low effort level means that things may not get done, will take ages, and frustration may move in due to lack of progress. Too much effort and you crash out with a setback again.

It's rather like checking a temperature in an oven. Too little heat, the dish is undercooked; too much heat, and the dish burns. An effort scale guides the balance of your activity to prevent a pacing disaster.

Rate the effort level of an activity on the scale overleaf:

Effort Scale for Pacing Activities and Goals

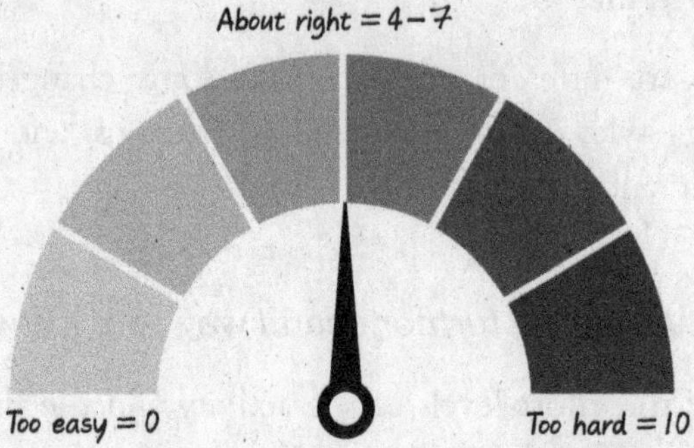

Give an effort level to the activities you pace. If your score is between four and seven, this is the balanced range of effort to succeed.

If effort level on the scale is:

3 or less	experiment further and spend more time on the activity **and/or** more speed;
8 or more	reduce it with more breaks **and/or** shorter time for activity.

Create and use a Daily Pacing Plan

You could create a Daily Pacing Plan like the one on page 140 to guide you and to balance and pace your activities. The guidelines below will help you to fill it in:

In the first column, list some of your daily activities.

In the Good day (second) and **Bad day (third) columns**, write down how long it typically takes to do each activity in minutes on a good day and a bad day. If there is a difference in these two figures, these activities need to be paced.

In the fourth column, write the number of minutes that you could **realistically** carry out that specific activity every day, without an increase in pain, stiffness and tiredness.

In the fifth column, write down the number of times you could repeat the activity.

In the final column, the effort scale level, write down the effort level for each activity. To do this, see more about the effort scale found after Razia's example here.

In the last column, enter **effort meter levels**, with the level to be between four to seven for the activity.

DAILY PACING PLAN

Activity Example to guide you: Weeding in garden	**Good day time plan mins** Spend 15 mins	**Bad day time plan** Spend 5 mins	**Everyday plan mins** Do 10 mins	**Times per day** 3 times per day	**Effort scale level (see effort meter)** 0 = none 10 = too much effort 5/10

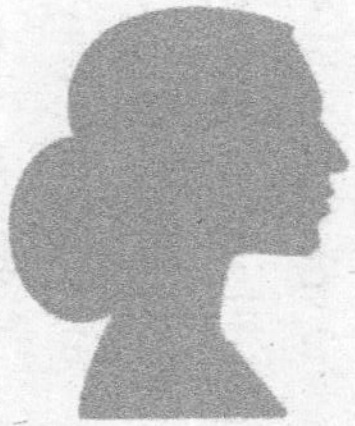

RAZIA'S DAILY PACING PLAN

Activity	Good day	Bad day	Everyday plan	Times per day	Effort scale level (0–10)
Standing and cooking	10 mins	5 mins	7 mins	5	6
Lying down for rest	15 mins	65 mins	25 mins	2	1
Walking	5 mins	2 mins	3 mins	4	5–6

What Razia found out . . .

Razia found she could do more activity **if** she factored in ten minutes of breathing and relaxation before she prepared the family meal.

She rewarded herself with a hot chocolate and a sit outside in the sunshine afterwards, then did another seven minutes in the kitchen. As it became easier to spend seven minutes in the kitchen for five times a day, she gradually increased her activity levels. She did this by increasing the amount of time she spent standing and the number of times she did jobs in the kitchen every day. She reduced the time in the day spent resting too, so helping her to build stamina and fitness in a paced way. Small footsteps built into a longer journey of change.

CREATE YOUR OWN DAILY PACING PLAN

- Have a go at creating your own pacing plan of daily activities.
- After one week, review how you are doing and decide if you could make some small steady

increases to your activity levels by increasing the time you spend doing them and reducing time resting.

- Notice whether you are feeling any of the benefits that come from pacing. **For example, less tired**. To remind yourself of what to look for, it might help to go back to the positive impacts that are listed earlier in this chapter.
- Make sure you let other people know about your plans, achievements and the rewards you plan.

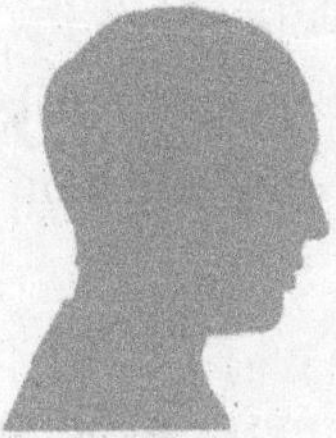

Jim's experience: it made a big difference to get Anne on board.

Jim wanted to change his overactive style of pacing, as he frequently rated his effort-level scale at eight, especially when he was working in the garden. He planned to give himself more breaks in his work routine and asked Anne to help him. They agreed that she would call him for a drink or a piece of fruit every thirty minutes and get Jim to have a five- to ten-minute break each time. Anne was glad to know how to help and be useful, and Jim was pleased that he was able to make some changes to his pacing style. Jim felt less tired, and now rated his effort-level score in the garden to scale six. Anne was surprised when Jim suggested that they go and see a movie later that day. Jim enjoyed this reward for the changes he had made, and he felt less sore and tired even though he had made progress in the garden.

Helpful pacing also needs **balanced thinking** that helps to focus the balance of time spent on an activity and rest periods or breaks. This thinking helps you keep up the activities which you value and are part of goals that you want to do either by yourself and with others. It is a really tricky skill to learn and use, yet makes a positive difference to being more active, sleep and pain itself.

Try to be aware of:

1. Thoughts like 'must' or 'should'; replace these with ***'could'***. For example, instead of thinking 'I must get it all done today', try thinking 'I could choose to pace, do it in stages over two or more days.'
2. Thinking that all the jobs must get done today. Watch for the unrealistic unhelpful 'all or nothing' thinking styles that are not helpful. It is not giving in, ***except*** to pain!

➔: page 246

Self-check on progress

What will help me to make progress?

This is the time to think about what will help you to succeed in changing your pacing style. These tips are from other people with pain who have tried them.

- **USE A TIMER:** Time your activities and stop using pain and tiredness as your guide. For example, some people use a timer on their mobile phones or a kitchen timer so that the alarm goes off to tell them it's time for a break.
- **PRIORITISE:** Think about what needs doing today, tomorrow and next week. People with pain often realise that the way they think about activities is unhelpful. Thoughts like 'I must get this all done now' lead to an overactive pacing style. Rather than thinking 'This must be done within the next day or so', try thinking 'I might get all this done this week.'
- **USE EFFORT LEVEL SCALE and AIM FOR BALANCE:** Get the effort level right and build in rest periods; for example, have a refreshing drink, listen to music, do breathing activities, talk with a friend or colleague. Making the rest period enjoyable means you are more likely to put in a break and look forward to it.

- **SET GOALS:** Everything is achievable given the right tools and length of time to complete the task. Set short- and long-term goals.
- **INVOLVE OTHERS:** Let them know what you are doing and why, get them to lend a hand, have some fun and plan a reward.
- **USE AN EFFORT LEVEL SCALE:** Use this to plan your activities like the one on page 138.

WORKING OUT WHAT WILL HELP YOU TO SUCCEED

Now that you have some ideas to help progress with pacing skills, have a go and complete the following activity.

Three things that will help me to pace better are:

1. ______________________________

   ____

   ____

2. ______________________________

   ____

   ____

3. ______________________________

   ____

   ____

One pacing change that I will try next week is:

____

____

Chapter summary

Tick the areas that were most helpful for you.

- ❑ Pacing is the key daily skill to improve all parts of your life. Identifying your pacing style and making changes helps you to find ways to balance activities and build in breaks.
- ❑ Over time this can help you do and achieve more with fewer setbacks.
- ❑ If you are underactive, steadily pace yourself towards more activity. If you are overactive, you need to plan and use more rest times and relaxation.
- ❑ Plan each day around what is important to achieve. Priorities are a vital part of pacing skills.
- ❑ Explore the effort and speed that you need to perform your activities, using the effort scale as a guide. Adjust levels to ensure you pace in a balanced way.
- ❑ Experiment with a Daily Plan regularly to find a balance between activities and rest or relaxation breaks and be prepared to fine-tune your pacing.

- ❑ Reward yourself often, especially for balancing pacing and your successes.

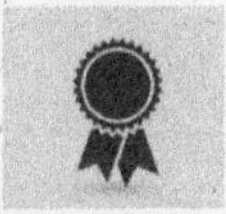

- ❑ Other areas ______________________________
____
____

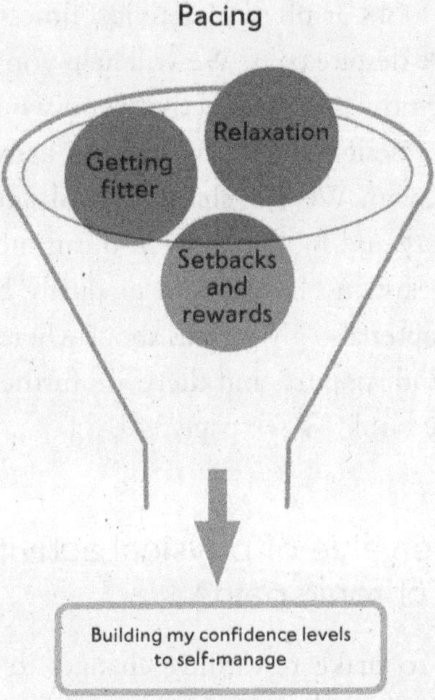

7

Being fitter and staying active

What this chapter covers

This chapter looks at physical activity, fitness and ways to be more active despite pain. We will help you explore what you are doing now and what activity you would like to do. Our bodies are designed to move and stay active, even if we have chronic pain. We will share more about the value of physical activity and look at how you can increase activity and exercise, sustain changes and gradually build up over time. This chapter also gives ideas about where to find more information and support, and there are further resources at the end of the book →: page 349.

What is the value of physical activity in managing chronic pain?

It is possible to make rewarding changes to your activity levels easily, safely and without increasing your pain. Being fitter and more physically active has lots of benefits, and research shows that exercise and activity help with managing moods, like anger and depression, improving concentration, reducing setbacks and improving sleep. Being active helps people achieve their day-to-day and longer-term goals. Gentle physical activity is good even on bad pain days as it helps the brain, the body and the pain networks to cope better.

Let's explore the issues Razia and Mo have with being more active.

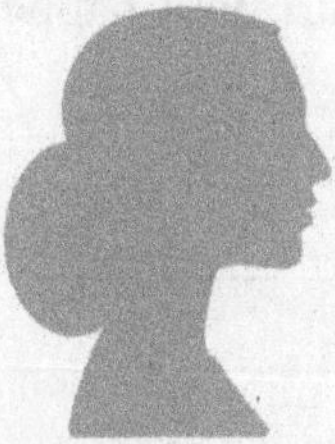

Razia struggles to cope with pain and stiffness, especially when the pain levels are high. She says, 'I try to rest until the pain settles, which often takes a couple of days.' This means 'I get so little done in the house; I feel weak and tired just standing to cook for Ali and Yousef and Hassan's parents.' Razia finds her pain and stiffness very unpredictable. It's tricky to plan her days, pace her activities, get jobs done and enjoy time with the children. Razia rests as much as possible to try and save her energy, manage her stiffness and lessen her pain, but this doesn't seem to be helping.

WHAT DO YOU THINK ABOUT RAZIA'S CURRENT ACTIVITY LEVEL?

Is Razia doing TOO MUCH, TOO LITTLE or JUST RIGHT? Circle what you think of Razia's activity and the reasons why.

What do you think might happen in the long term for Razia?

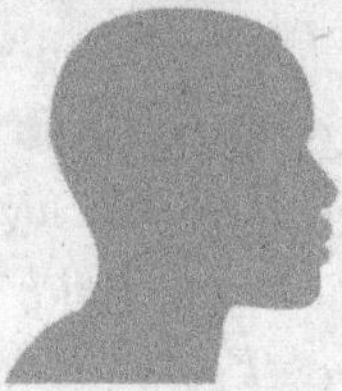

Mo is not able to pursue his hobbies, like cycling on Saturdays, any more, so he can't join in the weekly bike events. He wants to return to canoeing with his friends, but the pain in his neck and shoulder is just too bad. Now he spends most days resting in his room. He only goes out a couple of times a week to the food takeaway and to see his solicitor. He realises that he has lost friends, fitness, strength and stamina, and that there is much less fun and pleasure in his life. 'I am so stuck and limited.'

WHAT DO YOU THINK ABOUT MO'S CURRENT ACTIVITY LEVEL?

Is Mo doing TOO MUCH, TOO LITTLE or JUST RIGHT? Circle what you think of Mo's activity and the reasons why.

What do you think might happen in the long term for Mo?

____

____

How **confident** are you in your ability to do some physical activity?

0 1 2 3 4 5 6 7 8 9 10

Not at all confident — Extremely confident

Some useful things to know about physical activity

Research provides advice on the benefits of physical activity and the best types of activity and exercise.

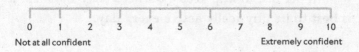

Top six benefits

1. Done on a regular basis, physical activity helps reduce the chances of heart disease, brain strokes, diabetes and dementia.
2. Being physically active helps maintain a healthy weight.
3. Fitness makes everyday tasks like going up and down stairs, getting washed, getting dressed, cooking and driving easier.
4. Increasing activity and doing something you enjoy improves confidence.
5. Physical activity reduces feelings of depression and anxiety, and helps manage anger and frustration.
6. Being physically and mentally active during the day improves sleep.

Do you know how much physical activity a person needs? It turns out that to help keep a balanced body and brain **it is best to be physically active every day**.

Types of activity that give benefits

Over a week, adults should aim to be active for a total of 150 minutes (2½ hours) of moderate intensity activity in bouts of 10 minutes or more. Moderate intensity means that you can still talk while exercising, you feel a little warmer and your heart beats faster. You can feel it beat in your chest, helping the heart muscle to become fitter and stronger.

Use SMART goals →: page 115 to build up from where you are now to thirty minutes of moderate physical activity on at least five days a week; for example, by walking, swimming or dancing.

Another option (with the same benefits) is to do seventy-five minutes of vigorous intense activity spread across the week. You can mix moderate and vigorous intense activity. Vigorous intensity means that more effort is needed, so the activity should be faster or harder, and you will feel much warmer, breathe quicker and harder, your heart will beat more rapidly and you will also find it quite difficult to carry on talking.

Adults should do exercises that increase muscle strength at least twice a week. This means making your muscles work so that they feel tight and hard when you touch them. Activities that strengthen muscles include using the stairs or doing exercises with weights, for example, a can of beans. Many parks have free equipment that helps with strength and fitness – have you checked out your local park? For more ideas on how to strengthen your body, look at the Resources at the end of the book.

Note: If you have chest pains or struggle for breath when you are physically active, you should discuss any changes you are planning to make with your doctor first.

The good news is that becoming fitter improves heart and mind health especially, lessens the impact of chronic pain, and helps achieve more and live well despite the pain.

Now that you know about the recommended levels of physical activity, do you think that Mo and Razia are doing enough?

How do you think they could build some physical activity into their daily and weekly routines SMARTly? →: page 115.

____

____

Understanding more about your physical activity now

Keeping a Physical Activity Diary

Let's find out more about your physical activity levels at the moment. A good starting point for this is a Physical Activity Diary. There is a diary you can use →: page 161, or you can use an online version.

TRACKING ACTIVITIES USING A PHYSICAL ACTIVITY DIARY

Use the diary to:

- Write down all the times you were physically active or you moved around doing tasks. It's a good idea to try and do this for more than one day, because your activity levels are likely to vary.
- Make sure you note down even if you were active for a few minutes, because even ten minutes of moderate activity can affect your fitness.
- Shade in the boxes for the hours when you were asleep, write down when and where you were resting, e.g. 2 to 3 p.m. sleep in chair, lounge.
- Write down when you were physically active and for how many minutes each time, for example write 'walking five mins', 'ironing fifteen mins' or 'going to the shops thirty mins'.

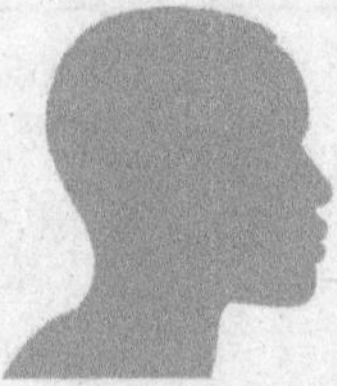

This is what Mo found when he looked at his **Physical Activity Diary**:

MO'S PHYSICAL ACTIVITY DIARY

Day, time and activity	Day + activity + minutes of activity **Monday**	Day + activity + minutes of activity **Tuesday**	Day + activity + minutes of activity **Wednesday**
6 a.m.	Sleeping – bedroom	Sleeping – bedroom	Sleeping – bedroom
7 a.m.	Sleeping	Sleeping	Sleeping
8 a.m.	Sleeping	Sleeping	Sleeping
9 a.m.	Sleeping	Sleeping	Sleeping
10 a.m.	Sleeping	Sleeping	Sleeping
11 a.m.	On the internet	Got up, had a shower, got dressed: ***fifteen minutes***	Watching TV – bedroom
12 p.m.	Sat and had a cup of tea with Mum and Dad	Lay on my bed for a rest	Looked on the internet for the local bike events
1 p.m.	Sleeping	Spoke on the phone with my solicitor – arranged an appointment	Walked to get fish and chips: ***ten minutes***

2 p.m.	Sat reading my canoeing magazine	Walked ***twenty minutes*** to the shop and back	Prayers with my dad
3 p.m.	Sleeping; chair in lounge	Read the paper	Dad took me to see the solicitor: walking ***fifteen minutes***
4 p.m.	Stood and ironed my clothes: ***thirty minutes***	Lay on the bed for a rest	Had a shower
5 p.m.	Watched a film in my room	Had a catch-up with what my friends are doing on social media	Argued with Mum and Dad over staying in my room so much
6 p.m.	Sleeping	Lay down on my bed as the pain was really bad	Lay on bed
7 p.m.	Sleeping	Lay on bed	Lay on bed
8 p.m.	Had a meal downstairs with Mum and Dad; walked about house: ***fifteen minutes***	Ordered a takeaway	Watched a film in my bedroom
9 p.m.		Went downstairs as takeaway had arrived: ***ten minutes***	Spoke to my friend on phone; he called about a cycle event
10 p.m.	Watched the news	Sleeping up in bedroom	Watched the news
11 p.m.	Lay on the bed and had a look at jobs online	Sleeping	Sleeping
12 a.m.	Sleeping	Sleeping	Sleeping

1 a.m.	Woke up having a nightmare	Sleeping	Sleeping
2 a.m.	Sleeping	Sleeping	Woke up in pain
3 a.m.	Lay awake in bed due to knee pain		Lay awake in bed unable to sleep due to pain and worries about money
4 a.m.	Sleeping	Sleeping	Sleeping
5 a.m.	Sleeping		Watched a film as couldn't get back to sleep

How many minutes of activity can you find that Mo recorded?

Mo discovered from his Physical Activity Diary his patterns of physical activity in his day. He was shocked at how much time he spent indoors, either on his computer, lying down, sleeping, reading or watching films. The diary showed him the areas where change might be possible so that he could get fitter, gain confidence and do more. From his diary entries Mo realised that on the days when he was more active, he felt more cheerful, his knee didn't feel so stiff and he slept better at night. These discoveries helped Mo to think about the benefits of becoming more active and setting some activity goals.

Physical Activity Diary – have a go at completing the table below

To help you understand your current activity levels and where to make changes, fill in your diary for a few typical days and review your entries. You may find that some activities are more helpful and enjoyable. Other activities may be more of a challenge at the moment, so it may be helpful to break them down into small chunks and build up slowly; things will get easier over time with practice. These same questions can guide your thinking and suggest ways in which you might change your daily physical activities.

PHYSICAL ACTIVITY DIARY: MY TYPICAL DAY

Day, time and activity	e.g. **Monday** **walked** to see friend: **ten minutes**	Day + activity + minutes of activity	Day + activity + minutes of activity
6 a.m.			
7 a.m.			
8 a.m.			
9 a.m.			
10 a.m.			

11 a.m.			
12 p.m.			
1 p.m.			
2 p.m.			
3 p.m.			
4 p.m.			
5 p.m.			
6 p.m.			
7 p.m.			
8 p.m.			
9 p.m.			
10 p.m.			
11 p.m.			
12 a.m.			
1 a.m.			
2 a.m.			
3 a.m.			
4 a.m.			
5 a.m.			

REVIEW YOUR PHYSICAL ACTIVITY DIARY

Take a look at what you have written in your diary and answer these questions:

1. From the Physical Activity Diary, how many minutes/hours did I spend physically active each day?

Day 1 ____________________________________

____

Day 2 ____________________________________

____

2. How many minutes/hours did I spend lying, resting or sitting down? This includes reading, sleeping or on a computer.

Day 1 ____________________________________

____

Day 2 ____________________________________

____

3. What kinds of activities seemed to help my pain, stiffness, mood and sleep?

____

____

4. Is there anything I could do differently?

____

____

If you are not sure, think about one or two changes that would be easy to make. This might be walking the dog twice a day, cleaning the bath or shower twice a week, taking a daily walk to the shop, standing to watch the football match.

Worries about doing more physical activity

You may have some worries about doing more activity or exercise. This is very common. People with pain, like Razia, often worry that physical activity will make their pain worse. They think that if their muscles or joints ache afterwards, this could be causing more damage or harm.

Some people, like Mo, have little or no motivation to increase their physical activity because they already feel too tired and weak. Not everyone knows how much or what physical activity to do, or where to go for help and support.

Think about your barriers to becoming more physically active right now and finish the sentence below:

The things that are getting in the way of me being more physically active are

____

____

If you aren't sure what to write, use the list below. Tick the points that relate to you and your situation at the moment:

❑ I don't know where to start.

❑ I don't know how much activity is enough.

❑ I'm not sure what the benefits of activity or fitness are.

❑ I hate exercise.

❑ The exercises the physio gave me made the pain worse.

- ❑ I can't speak when I am walking.
- ❑ I get scared when my heart beats faster.
- ❑ Pain stops me doing more.
- ❑ I don't like getting sweaty.
- ❑ There's nowhere to shower and change when I get to work.
- ❑ I can't afford a gym pass.
- ❑ It makes me so tired.
- ❑ I don't know what to wear.
- ❑ I have no one to walk with me.
- ❑ Other reasons.

____

____

____

____

Tools that can support you to make changes

Five Key Steps to help increase Physical Activity

Step 1: Make it enjoyable

- Choose enjoyable activities, such as taking a walk to watch the birds, or listening to music while gently stretching.
- Dance around the kitchen to your favourite song.

Step 2: Make it sociable

- Get the whole family involved – tell others what you are trying to do.
- Play with the kids – tumble in the leaves, build a snowman, splash in a puddle, throw a ball.
- Volunteer to plant or care for a community garden.

Step 3: Make it easy to fit into daily or weekly routines

- Do push-ups against a bedroom wall.
- Stand up to watch part of a football match; walk on the spot if you like to keep moving.
- If the kids are playing football, or are in a playground, walk around the pitch or park.
- Do stretches, exercises, or pedal a stationary bike while watching television.

- Stand up when you are using your mobile, or even walk around outside.

Step 4: Try out new things

- Try an exercise class at the local leisure centre. Yoga, Pilates and t'ai chi all improve balance and reduce the chance of falls, as well as helping with concentration and body relaxation. Many such centres have classes especially for people who are older or who are starting to exercise after illness or accidents. Check out your local public leisure or activity centre website for details.
- Exercise to a new workout video or yoga app.

Step 5: Build up slowly and steadily

- Walk the dog a minute or two longer each day; do an extra lap around the block every week.
- Get off the bus a stop earlier than normal and walk to work; do this for one week and then gradually get off the bus a stop earlier still, and so on.

What do you think *you* could try from the five steps list above?

What other ideas have you got?

What ideas have other people suggested to you?

Self-check on progress

What will help me to increase my activity, make progress?

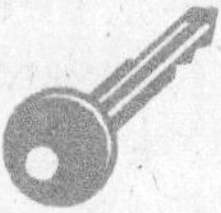

Goal setting and pacing skills: pages 110 and 125 are the tools you need to become more active. Remember to build in rewards as you achieve each step of your goal and build up steadily over a period of time. Have a look at the other chapters in this book on Balancing daily activities through pacing and Reaching goals and creating rewards to help you get started.

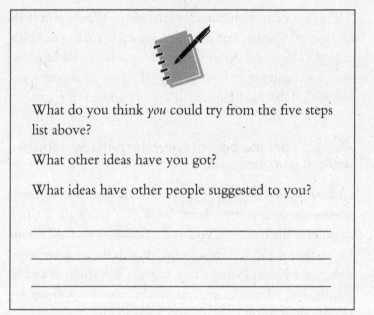

Plan your day with times for relaxation or rest and periods of physical activity. For example, get up to make yourself a cup of coffee, and do some stretching exercises while you wait for the kettle to boil. It may take a bit of experimenting to find the right balance of activity and rest for you.

How do I get the benefits of more physical activity without pain setbacks?

Gradually increase your physical activity levels over time. Start with your current level; so, if you can walk for five minutes at the moment, you might decide to increase this to five minutes and fifteen seconds. As this distance becomes easier to achieve, increase to five and a half minutes and so on, so that, after perhaps four weeks, you are walking for ten minutes. Small changes over time add up.

Remember that it is normal to get some mild muscle or joint ache when you start or increase activity. These aches do not mean you are causing more damage or harm to your body; in fact, they are a good sign that your muscles are getting stronger and your joints are loosening up. As you do more regular activity, these aches and pains will settle down.

Some people may benefit from a structured traditional exercise programme that aims to improve stamina, muscle strength, balance and coordination or flexibility. A physiotherapist, personal trainer or health advisor would be happy to discuss your needs and help you to confidently move forward.

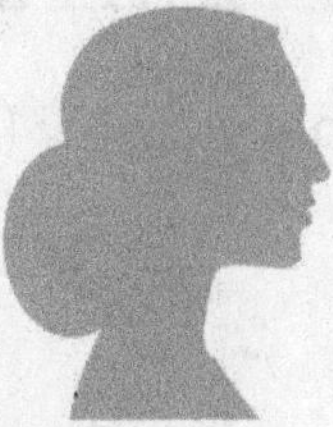

Razia struggled to be more active. She really feared it would make her pain worse. Her mother-in-law asked her to start walking in the park with her. Razia reluctantly agreed to try as she had just found out about pacing skills. She found that by walking every day, with a short rest period at the café, she was soon able to walk for ten minutes at a time. Razia noticed her muscles ached less than she predicted and her confidence to be more active grew.

My action plan, to create and do a SMART activity ➔: page 115 or fitness goal.

____

____

____

____

____

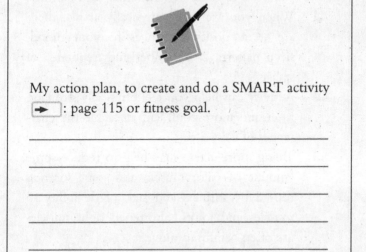

Chapter summary

Tick the areas that were most helpful for you.

- ❑ Realising that being more physically active has many health benefits.
- ❑ Everyone can benefit from more physical activity in their lives, even if they have health problems.
- ❑ It is possible to do more physical activity despite pain, and to cause benefit rather than harm.
- ❑ When you are more physically active, there are some positive changes to your mood, sleep pattern, and number and frequency of setbacks.
- ❑ Activity can help you feel physically stronger, fitter and more confident to tackle the challenges of daily life.
- ❑ Being more active may help to reduce some amount of pain, muscle and joint soreness caused by stiffness and lack of flexibility in muscles and joints. Shortened tight muscles are often painful to move.

- ❑ There are five steps to build fitness slowly and steadily, and the benefits soon become noticeable to you and others.
- ❑ Choose something fun, enjoyable and sociable, such as walking groups or t'ai chi classes.
- ❑ More personal physical activity programmes, involving courses or groups or health fitness trainers can be designed around you and your needs.
- ❑ Other things I valued from this chapter

____

____

____

8

Relaxing more easily

What this chapter covers

This chapter is about learning to relax the body and mind. Relaxation, along with other soothing and calming activities, can help manage pain well. The chapter focuses on how learning to relax can change the impact of pain. There are ideas on how to unwind both the body and the mind, how to practise letting go of tension, and overcoming any barriers to being more relaxed.

Why relaxation can help manage pain better

Relaxation is more than simply sitting still and doing nothing. You can be very tense while sitting or lying still. For instance, when sitting you could be watching a horror movie on TV or playing an exciting computer game; or you could be lying in bed thinking about the frustrations of the day.

When you relax, the tension or hardness in your muscles is reduced. Reducing tension or making the muscles feel softer can make you feel calm and comfortable. Relaxation also means allowing the mind to become less active, giving it a break, which can rapidly slow down often quite emotional thoughts. Relaxation skills can be very useful for anyone, especially those who are living with chronic pain.

HOW DO YOU KNOW WHEN YOU'RE RELAXED?

What do you notice about yourself when you feel relaxed?	**What do you notice about yourself when you feel stressed or worried?**
Tick those that apply to you:	Tick those that apply to you:
Warm	Shallow, fast breathing
Heavy or light in the body	Muscular tension/hardness
Slow, controlled breathing	'Clouded' mind
Less muscular tension	Poor concentration and memory
Clearer mind, more alert	Difficulty making decisions
Good concentration and memory	More pain
Less pain	Racing or repeated thoughts
Mood – lighter and brighter	Mood – low or worried moods
Others?	Others?

Slowing the body and mind helps them to become more aware of ways to manage pain well.

Regular practice of a relaxation technique over a number of weeks/months is needed so that you can learn the difference between contracted and relaxed muscles and 'retrain the brain' to unwind tense body areas and muscles.

How can relaxation help with chronic pain?

When muscles are tense, it can cause pain, or make existing pain worse. For instance, many people find that their shoulders or neck hurt after a stressful day. This pain is often due to tense muscles and altered body positions, which might be held tight for a long time.

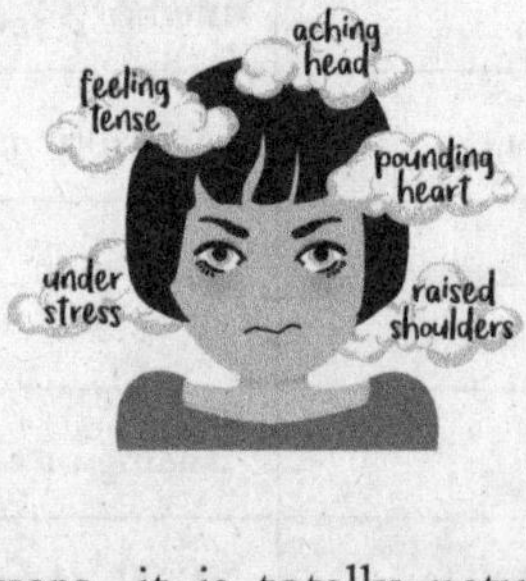

When pain is severe, it is totally natural to tense up in response to it, as when anxious. Tightened muscles, gritting one's teeth, a tense tight jaw or shoulders, all add to pain. Learning to notice tension early, and reduce it, can be very useful. Being relaxed will help you manage pain more successfully. Relaxation can give you a break from tension in the middle of a difficult, possibly frustrating day. It can remind you not to rush or 'overdo it' and improve your use of pacing skills →: page 125. It is about 'retraining the brain' through regular relaxation practices over a few weeks/months. You will discover and feel the difference within your body; between it (especially the muscles) being tight or tense and relaxed. This, in turn, helps to lessen some pain.

Useful things to know about relaxation

Relaxation is a skill that takes practice to learn and some people find it easier than others. It is a positive activity you can do every day, anywhere and anytime, even in the middle of a severe setback →: page 319. Relaxation can make setbacks less likely; and if they do happen, they can be less intense, and settle down more quickly.

There are many different ways to relax, so experiment to find those that work best for you. Some people find that visualising relaxing images, such as a walk in the country or on a beach, is the most calming for them. For others, focusing on different patterns of breathing is most useful. This is because unhelpful breathing patterns can cause a range of symptoms – tiredness, neck pain, breathlessness, anxiety, tingling in the hands, aching jaw, teeth grinding, etc., and these worsen pain. Regular practice of a 'new habit' of 'diaphragm or belly breathing' can help, and explore Resources ➔: page 357.

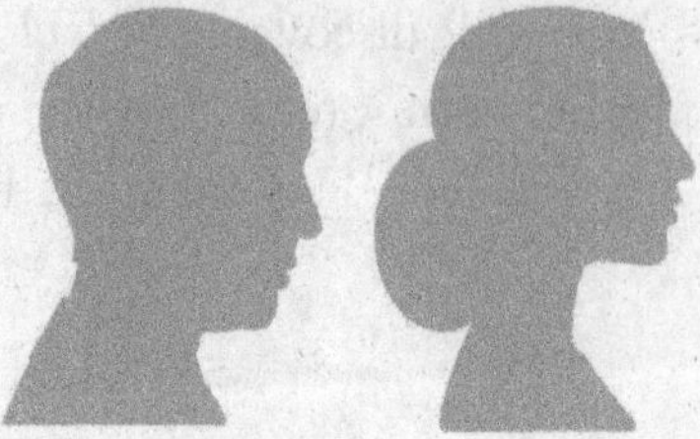

Jim and Razia found relaxation a valuable coping skill to help manage pain more successfully. Jim found it helped him pace the day well and he slept better at night as he felt calmer. His partner Anne agreed that he seemed less bothered and irritable as a result. Razia found that relaxation gave her a brief break to recharge her energy levels when she had a moment to herself.

How well do you relax now?

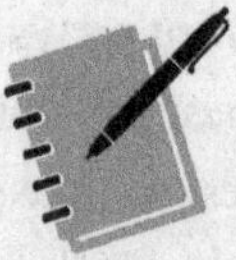

Here are a few ideas that may help you to relax.

Tick three choices as a start point, and try to pace them into your daily life:

What can help you relax at present?

- ❑ Simple breathing patterns like 'belly breathing'.
- ❑ Concentrating on reducing tension in various parts of the body.
- ❑ Self-hypnosis.
- ❑ Sitting in a beautiful garden, smelling the flowers, listening to nature.
- ❑ Imagining pleasant images or pictures.
- ❑ Listening to a relaxation recording.
- ❑ A nice long soak in a warm bathtub.
- ❑ Listening to a favourite piece of music.
- ❑ Exercise programmes, like yoga, t'ai chi or Pilates.
- ❑ Attending a local relaxation or mindfulness group.
- ❑ Being somewhere comfortable, soothing and safe.
- ❑ Recorded sounds of nature, like sea waves or birds singing.
- ❑ Focusing on a candle or looking at a beautiful picture.
- ❑ Pleasant smells, such as aromatherapy oils.
- ❑ Other – write them down:

____

____

____

What makes you feel relaxed?

Write or draw your ideas in your notebook or on a tablet/ phone. Then try to make them into a SMART goal and see if this helps you to practise them → : page 110.

Are there different ways to relax through the day? Sometimes activities like knitting or craftwork or completing a model – in which you are both enjoying yourself and engaging the mind and body – are relaxing. It can help to engage in activities such as making things, giving things and sharing things. These activities help calm and quieten the mind and allow space to refocus on living well in the here and now.

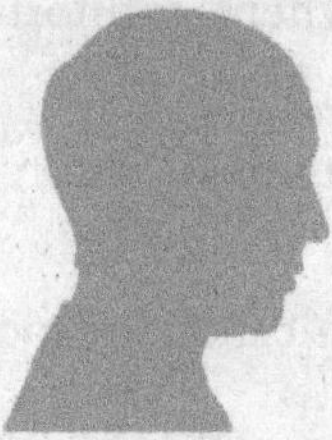

Jim found out that Anne was into knitting, as it helped to take her mind away from her breathing problems, making her feel less frustrated, calmer in herself. She suggested to Jim that he try it too; 'It sort of soothes me,' she said. Anne needed Jim to help with making knitted flower shapes for a local festival event. He reluctantly agreed;

initially, though, only for two weeks. Three months later, he observed: 'Who would have thought I could be so creative: a whole bunch of knitted flowers and vegetables! I am going to try model toys next.'

Practising relaxation and tools that can support your relaxation skills

How to unwind and practise relaxation

These are two useful approaches that people with pain find helpful.

Time-out relaxation

For a 'time-out' relaxation session, set aside about twenty to thirty minutes. Making time to practise and focus on relaxing will help you learn how to relax fully and deeply. When you first learn a relaxation technique, being in a quiet, comfortable place can help. Lie down on a bed or mat, or sit in your most comfortable chair. Try to find a time when you are unlikely to be disturbed. If you wish, a partner or friend could do the relaxation session with you. Or you may prefer to do it alone. Listening to a recording or going to a class can be called 'time-out' relaxation. There are lots of relaxation apps or online recordings available to buy. (**Note**: If you plan to use a relaxation recording, don't use it while driving or operating machinery!) Try and look at your relaxation sessions as part of your treatment, viewing it in the same way as a daily activity programme. Explore the Resources suggested at the end of this book →: page 357.

Quick relaxation

As well as using a 'time-out' technique, you can start to use relaxation in everyday situations. As soon as you notice any tension or hardness build in your muscles, practise 'letting go' of the tension, 'breathe it gently away' and relax. When you have had a bit more practice, you can use relaxation and breathing in more stressful situations – for instance, when you feel yourself getting angry or frustrated.

You can also practise 'scanning'. This means checking your body for tension by noticing your feet, your legs, your knees, your hips, your abdomen, your chest, your shoulders, your neck, your head, your face and your jaw. As you notice any tension let it go, release it from you. As a tip, start from toes and work upwards, 'letting go' of your tension on the out-breath.

Let go in the feet ... then in the legs ...

You can also observe your breathing, and remember to breathe calmly and comfortably. As you breathe in, your tummy should rise a little; then rest back as you breathe

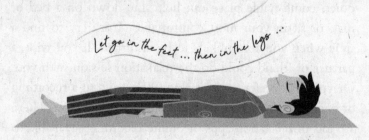

out. Don't force things, as this may make you feel a little 'light-headed'.

Use 'reminders' – for example, put a sticker on the fridge or on your mirror, and check for tension each time you see the sticker.

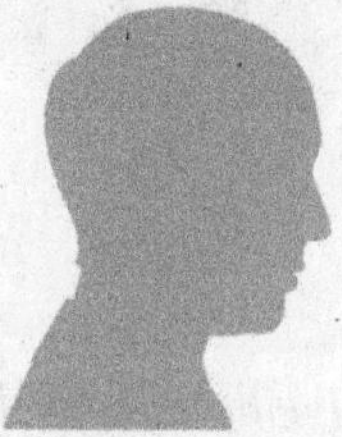

Jim put a reminder by the kettle to help him remember time for relaxation or calming soothing activities, like crosswords. After two weeks he found it had become natural to practise his relaxation and breathing twice daily and do a word puzzle every day, as well. Jim began to value his days and activities more, even when the pain was troublesome.

Problem-solving ideas when it is difficult to practise relaxation

It can be difficult to make time to practise relaxation without being disturbed. If you have a lot of demands on your time, you may need to be creative about when and how you fit in your relaxation. You may feel that you are the sort of person who 'just can't relax'. However, there is usually a way round these obstacles →: page 328.

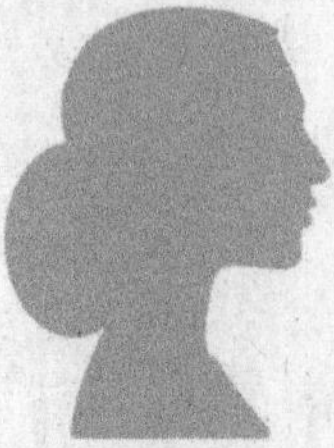

Razia experimented with times in the day that she could relax and found she could do ten minutes of gentle relaxation breathing after her morning and evening prayers. Everybody knew it was prayer time and did not disturb her. Adding it on to prayer times seemed 'worth a try and a good idea'. This helped Razia pace herself during the busy times getting the children ready and off to school.

You can use problem-solving skills →: page 327 to help you overcome barriers. Here are more ideas that might be helpful: tick ones to try.

- ❑ Try a regular appointment with yourself at a certain time of day.
- ❑ Let others know that you are not available at that time.
- ❑ Switch off your phone.
- ❑ Notice times in the day when you are least busy, or when people are least likely to call – experiment using those times for relaxation sessions.

- ❑ Perhaps make time and space when your children have gone to school, or your partner has gone out.
- ❑ You could practise your relaxation skills at times of the day when you are by yourself.
- ❑ Remind others (and yourself!), if you need to, that this is a daily treatment. You are not 'being lazy'; it is helping the body and brain to manage pain and pace itself better.
- ❑ If you find yourself feeling guilty about taking time out, check out unhelpful thinking →: page 242.

Using relaxation resources

When getting ready to listen to a relaxation recording, make sure the lights are dim and the temperature suits you. It may be difficult to find a position in which to lie down or sit comfortably. This does not mean that you can't benefit from the relaxation. At first, as soon as you start, you may want to fidget or cough, or you may get an itch or a fit of giggles. If so, feel free to change position, scratch or laugh! Use breathing exercises as a guide. On relaxation apps or downloads, you are often asked to breathe deeply and evenly.

Remember that you do not have to hold your breath to wait for the next instruction. See Resouces →: page 357.

Some people find that they have odd thoughts or images going through their minds when they start to learn to relax. This is quite normal and happens to most people. However, if you get a lot of really distressing thoughts or images after trying an exercise a few times, talk to a person skilled in relaxation therapy or talking therapy. There is usually a way to overcome such experiences.

Some people find that they fall asleep before the end of a session. This is not a problem, but, with more practice, you will probably find that you don't fall asleep. Then you will feel even more relaxed and refreshed at the end of the session.

Relaxation exercises can be fun, as well as helping you manage pain. They can give you a feeling of well-being and alertness without tension. This is particularly helpful if medication makes you drowsy. Some people do not initially enjoy learning relaxation skills, partly because they feel a loss of control. Try to find what works best for you: music, colour-focused relaxation or doing calming, soothing activities such as knitting, birdwatching, playing cards, using a mindfulness colouring book. Explore and try a few possibilities.

Who benefits from practising regular relaxation?

Nearly everybody can benefit from some form of relaxation. If you have had a recent severe mental illness or are experiencing ongoing post-traumatic stress disorder, get some advice from your mental health support team before starting. If you have any questions, make notes to share when you see your therapist or healthcare professional.

Self-check on progress

Learning to relax is a skill, which means it can take time to learn, and more practice means you get better at it. You may need to practise for several weeks consistently to help 'retrain the brain' before it starts to come more naturally. Keep a note of how often you do your relaxation practice and notice any benefits for your body, how you feel and think, and the impact it has on your pain. Try experimenting with different relaxation styles to see which ones seems to work best for you. Use the audio resources from the suggested links in Resources : page 357; many people with pain find them helpful.

Write the benefits of relaxation on the Five-Areas diagram overleaf.

Five Areas Tool: My Benefits of Relaxation

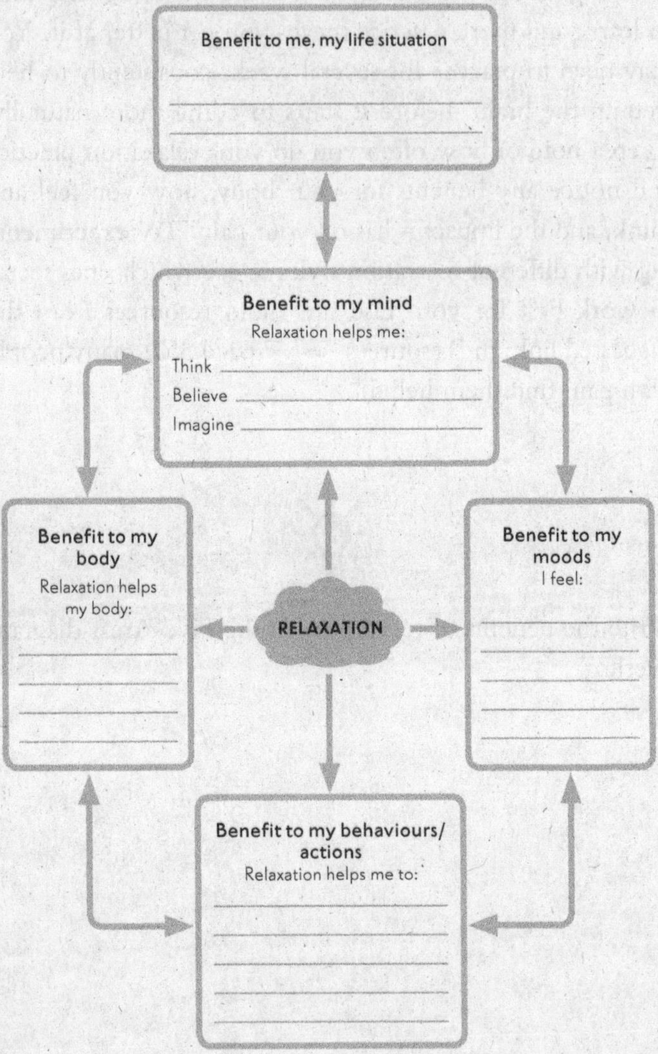

Chapter summary

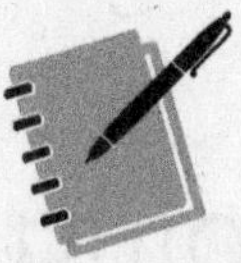

- Learning relaxation is a skill you can use to reduce bodily tension and stressful thinking. This also helps the brain manage pain better, as it unwinds and soothes the mind.
- Relaxation can help to turn down the volume of chronic pain and tension by helping to loosen the muscles and joints.
- There are different ways of relaxing, including time-out relaxation, quick relaxation and doing relaxing enjoyable activities such as knitting, painting, watching animals play, and so forth.
- Spotting barriers to doing relaxation practice and dealing with them means they interfere less with relaxation time and space.

9

Sleeping well

What this chapter covers

In this chapter we look at the common difficulties people experience when they are not sleeping well; whether it is too little sleep or oversleeping. We explain how pain and sleep can interfere with each other, and suggest some ways that you can understand and improve your sleep pattern.

What is the value of sleeping well in managing chronic pain?

Sleeping well with pain is possible, and it can help to lessen the way pain affects you from day to day ➔: page 6. These are the kinds of problems people can have with sleep:

- Difficulty getting off to sleep.
- Waking often.
- Problems dropping off again.
- Waking early in the morning and being unable to sleep again.
- Feeling tired, groggy and not refreshed on waking.

- Sleeping too much or for too long.
- Dropping off to sleep in the day.

For many people with chronic pain, there are some **extra problems** that can interfere with getting a good night's sleep.

SLEEP PROBLEM LIST USING THE FIVE-AREAS TOOL

Tick the extra problems other than pain that affect your sleep at the moment:

Bedroom or sleeping-place situation

❑ I can't get comfortable in bed.

❑ Partner's snoring problems getting worse.

❑ It is noisy in the house or outside.

Body symptoms

❑ I get cramp(s).

❑ I can't lie still.

❑ I've got restless legs.

❑ My medicines make me feel drowsy.

- ❑ My medicines make me feel too wide-awake.
- ❑ Medicines to help me sleep make me feel 'hungover' and drowsy the next day.
- ❑ My snoring problem is getting worse.
- ❑ I wake up because of pain or nightmares.

Moods and thoughts

- ❑ My mood goes down in the night, and I end up feeling more miserable.
- ❑ I feel tense and it's harder to get back to sleep once I've woken up.
- ❑ I end up with my problems and worries going round and round in my head.
- ❑ Time passes so slowly in the night and there's no one to talk to.

Behaviours/Actions

- ❑ I don't get enough activity in the day.
- ❑ I end up napping in the day.
- ❑ I did too much yesterday.

Other things you or others have noticed

____

The trouble with lack of good-quality sleep is that it can make us feel groggy, sleepy, tired, edgy and irritable the next day. It can also affect our concentration and memory, leaving us feeling worried about sleep problems and even causing difficulties at work or when doing life activities. Unfortunately, poor sleep can reduce your pain tolerance as well, so it's really worth seeing if you can improve things.

The good news is that disrupted sleep patterns can improve, even if you have chronic pain. Improved sleep can help reduce the amount of pain, and research shows that if you sleep well, even with pain, then your moods, tiredness and pain-related symptoms improve.

Useful things to know about sleep

How much sleep do you need?

Everyone is different in how much time they spend sleeping and how much sleep they need. When we are less active, we need less sleep, but we can feel more tired. Our need for sleep changes with age.

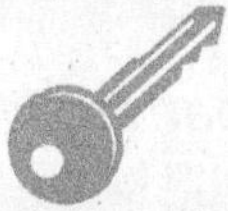

Useful facts, about the amount of sleep we need:

- A teenager usually needs about ten hours' sleep.
- At age forty to sixty, we usually need six to seven hours' sleep.

- At age sixty and older, we need only five to six hours' sleep.

You may have a clear idea of how much sleep you should get. Does it match what it says here? Yes? . . . No? . . . Maybe.

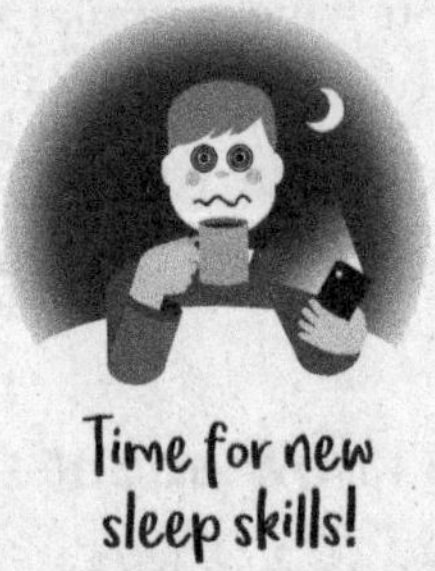
Time for new
sleep skills!

Understanding more about your sleep difficulties

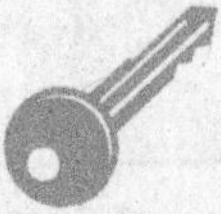

1. What is your sleep pattern like now?

Use these questions to find out about your sleep patterns at the moment:

1. How many hours' sleep do you get, on average, at night?

2. How many hours' sleep do you get, on average, during the day?
3. Do you feel you are getting enough sleep?
4. What things seem to affect how well you sleep? (Use the problem list, above, for ideas, and add your own experiences.)
5. What thoughts and worries do you have about your sleeping pattern?
6. Do you find that after you have slept, you feel bright and alive, ready to face the day?

Note: You may want to discuss with your doctor or pharmacist any concerns about your medicines and how they affect your sleep. Use the Guide to Safe Medicine Use →: page 377.

2. Keeping a sleep diary to track sleep patterns

Jim was worried about Anne's health, and everything he had to do to help her, coupled with his own pain, made it harder for him to sleep. He wanted to feel rested, less tired and anxious, and to sleep well, so he started by keeping a sleep diary. See his completed diary →: page 196.

A 'sleep diary' is a good starting point to improve sleep. It will help you to discover more about your sleep patterns at the moment. There is a blank diary you can use on →: page 198, or you can use an online version.

For a whole week, write down all the times you were asleep. It's helpful, also, to record where you were when you fell asleep; for example, you may have dropped off in front of the TV.

Make a record even if you just dozed off for a few minutes, because this can affect your sleep at night. Also record:

- Any medicines you have taken, which may affect your sleep.
- If you were worried or if you had any nightmares.
- If any pain or discomfort stopped you sleeping or woke you up.
- Anything else you noticed, e.g. having alcoholic drinks in an evening, eating late at night.

Here is Jim's sleep diary, for the first week. The shaded areas show when he was asleep.

JIM'S SLEEP DIARY

Time	Mon	Tue	Wed	Thu	Fri	Sat	Sun
6 a.m.							
7 a.m.							
8 a.m.							
9 a.m.							
10 a.m.							
11 a.m.							
12 p.m.							
1 p.m.							In the car
2 p.m.		Asleep in chair		1 hr in my chair			

3 p.m.							
4 p.m.	30 mins						
5 p.m.							
6 p.m.							
7 p.m.							
8 p.m.							
9 p.m.	Ate late supper	Asleep in chair					
10 p.m.							
11 p.m.					11.30 fell asleep in bed		Bed
12 a.m.		In bed	Bed	Anne had problems too		Bed	
1 a.m.							
2 a.m.	Bed						
3 a.m.			½ hour no sleep	½ hr no sleep			In chair
4 a.m.		Awake again					
5 a.m.							

Jim found out that he slept better when he hadn't dropped off in the day. Sleeping in a chair made him more uncomfortable and a bit grumpy when he woke up. He realised that some of the time he was awake in the night he was going over problems in his mind.

SLEEP DIARY

Fill this in for at least several days or a week and make a note of:

- Where you were when you were asleep – **shade the box in**.
- When you took medicines for pain or sleep.
- Whether anything seemed to keep you awake.

Time	Mon	Tue	Wed	Thu	Fri	Sat	Sun
6 a.m.							
7 a.m.							
8 a.m.							
9 a.m.							
10 a.m.							
11 a.m.							
12 p.m.							
1 p.m.							
2 p.m.							
3 p.m.							
4 p.m.							
5 p.m.							
6 p.m.							
7 p.m.							
8 p.m.							
9 p.m.							
10 p.m.							
11 p.m.							

12 a.m.							
1 a.m.							
2 a.m.							
3 a.m.							
4 a.m.							
5 a.m.							

Once you have filled in the diary for several days or a week, what do you notice? Make a note of any patterns, or things that seem to help.

What would you like to try to change? There are some ideas below.

Ideas for improving your sleep

1. Getting into a regular sleep pattern

We know that having a regular routine prior to bedtime can help children to sleep better. It can help adults too. Being 'in tune' with your body's natural rhythms, or 'biological clock', can make the sleep you have feel more satisfying, and make you feel more alert when you are awake.

To establish a sleep pattern, you could try out this technique, which has been shown to improve sleep:

1. First, think about how many hours of sleep you need. Remember, everyone is different, so try to think about how many hours you typically sleep when you have a decent night.
2. Next, decide what time you want to get up every morning.
3. Now, take away your sleep hours from your getting-up time. This is your new time to go to bed to sleep.
4. From now on, make sure that you go to bed at this time and get up at the same time every morning, regardless of how you have actually slept.

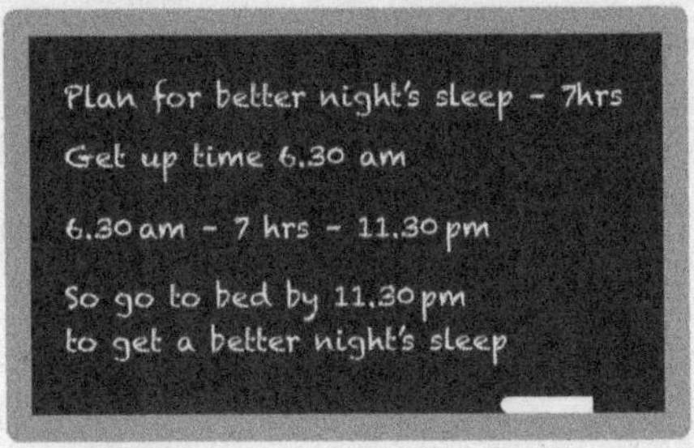

Plan for better night's sleep - 7hrs
Get up time 6.30 am
6.30 am - 7 hrs - 11.30 pm
So go to bed by 11.30 pm
to get a better night's sleep

Sticking to a regular sleep pattern can be a challenge if you haven't slept well, but it is worth persevering.

People with persistent pain, fatigue or other symptoms may need a rest during the day. If you do need to have a nap, choose the best time for you. You may find that if you sleep in the daytime for more than fifteen minutes it interferes with your night-time sleep. Therefore, try to make sure you have a very short nap and, if possible, try to avoid using your bedroom for naps, as napping could then become your night-time routine.

2. Having a regular winding-down routine

Here are some other ideas for ensuring you have a regular winding-down routine, soothing the body and mind to prepare for sleep.

Tick at least one that you could try out:

Food and drink

- ❑ Have a light snack, a milky drink or a herbal tea before you go to bed; perhaps have your own special mug for bedtime.
- ❑ Try to avoid caffeinated drinks several hours before bed.

Relaxation

- ❑ Have a relaxing bath or shower, maybe adding a calming aromatherapy-type oil.
- ❑ Avoid any hard physical activities for at least a few hours before bed, as it can take a while to get ready for sleep after an exercise session.
- ❑ Use relaxation techniques ➔: page 174 earlier in the evening.

- ❑ Use a 'quick relaxation' if you feel tense when you go to bed.
- ❑ Relaxing music may help some to get to sleep quicker.

Soothing the mind

- ❑ Have a 'worry'/'things to remember' notebook handy, so that you can make a note and put worries to one side to be dealt with the next day.
- ❑ Avoid stimulating your mind just before bed, e.g. don't watch an action movie or work, or read emails / social media late in the evening.

Helping your brain to link your bedroom with sleep

- ❑ Keep the bedroom for sleeping and sex.
- ❑ Avoid the use of screens, e.g. TV, mobile phones, tablets.
- ❑ If you have to have your phone with you at night, consider turning off alerts.
- ❑ Put your phone out of reach, dim the screen brightness, avoid checking it if you are awake during the night.

Medication

- ❑ If you take medicines at night, take them at the same time.
- ❑ If you have any questions about how your tablets affect your sleep, write them down in your notebook. Discuss them at your next appointment with the doctor who prescribes them →: page 377.

3. Preparing your bedroom

This is about being comfortable and getting ready to sleep well. Try to make sure you have low lighting and the temperature in the room is not too warm or too cold. A cooling fan can be helpful in warmer weather. Your mattress should be comfortable, and it may help to have an extra pillow to go between your knees, or behind your back. Try to make sure your bedroom is a clutter-free zone.

Things that you can do if you can't get to sleep

If you can't get to sleep, or you wake up in the night and can't get back to sleep, it can help to follow the suggestions below. These will help to prevent you from lying in bed awake for long periods.

- Get up, rather than lie there too long, e.g. after fifteen minutes.
- If possible, go into a different room and keep the lights fairly low.
- Remember to use your notebook to keep a record of things that are worrying you or write a 'to-do' list for the next day.
- Do something uninteresting if you are awake in the night, e.g. read something 'light'/listen to something calming (but not in your bed). It can help to get these ready in advance so that you know what to do.
- Avoid any temptation to switch on the TV.

- Practise quick relaxation skills [➔]: page 182.
- Go back to bed when you feel sleepy, but still try to get up at the usual time.

If you are restless, you may be worried about disturbing your partner, and this can make you feel more tense.

If you haven't talked about it already, try finding out how much you are disturbing them. Find out if they mind and what would help. You may need to try sleeping in separate rooms or separate beds for a while, until the problem has eased.

4. Dealing with worries and unhelpful thoughts

It is often the case that a restless mind keeps us awake at night. If you find that you lie in bed worrying or planning things, then try these tips:

- You're likely to be better at problem solving ([➔]: page 375) when you are supposed to be awake. You can make a time for yourself in the day when you can think things through properly. Earmark a proper 'worry half-hour' in the day; this leaves you free to get on with the rest of your day, and perhaps sleep better at night.
- Have a 'worries and things to remember' notebook. It can help to make a note of things you need to deal with.
- At night, tell yourself, 'I can think about that

tomorrow', make a note, and put it to one side. It can be difficult, but it gets easier with practice.

- You have probably noticed that 'trying hard' to go to sleep can be unhelpful. Worrying about not being asleep can keep you awake. If you have done everything reasonable to prepare for sleep, you will at least be fairly relaxed and able to rest your body.
- Try not to worry if you break your routine sometimes. If you've decided to do this on purpose, it can be easier to accept that you may not sleep so well.

5. Dealing with sleeping too much

Some people find that they are spending too much time asleep. There can be a number of reasons for this. Explore and plan an action that may help.

Take a look at the list and identify which ones may apply to you:

Medicines can cause drowsiness

Talk to your family doctor, as a whole range of medicines have this side-effect, including amitriptyline, nortriptyline, gabapentin, strong opioids, and some anti-depressants.

Snoring and short pauses in your sleep that leave you tired the next day, problems with concentration, falling asleep easily while doing tasks.

Talk to your GP / family doctor and explore more about sleep apnoea problems, especially if you have become very overweight. (For sleep apnoea information ➔: Resources on page 354.)

Sleeping because of boredom
Try to plan your day to occupy yourself and add why the activity is important – try out the Daily Activity Planner or ➔: page 364. Add pleasurable activities into your Daily Activity Plan.

Sleeping to avoid pain
Work out what is important to do or enjoyable in the day and actively incorporate them in your daily activity planner ➔: page 364.

Focus on things you value doing with people who are important to you. Then get started and try goal setting skills if that helps with using the Daily Activity Plan.

Sleeping due to low mood
Try to spend time outdoors, so that you get real daylight; this helps the sleep cycle clock. Increasing physical activity steadily may also help. Explore the chapter on Coping with low mood, depression and loss →: page 290; talk with your family doctor.

Mobile phones, tablets and sleep

If sleep is really important to you, the best advice is to stop using a mobile device in bed or for one to two hours before sleep. The brightness of the screen can stimulate your brain into thinking it is daytime!

- Turn off alerts.
- Put your phone out of reach.
- Dim the screen brightness setting.
- Set a lights-off/phone-off time.
- Use your phone to play a relaxation track, mindfulness exercise, music or podcast.
- Be bored for a while! Try distraction for ten minutes.
- Really can't face any of these as the first step? What else could you try?

What will help me to make progress?

Like Jim, you may find it helps to make an action plan to improve your sleep:

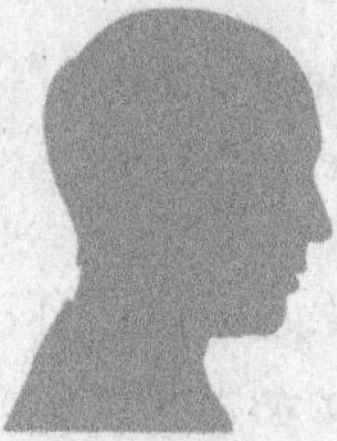

Jim chose and incorporated these things to do in his Daily Activity Plan:

- *Use some relaxation breathing before settling to sleep.*
- *Keep a notepad by the bed to write down all worries about jobs before sleep.*
- *Have lighter evening meals two hours earlier than usual.*
- *Avoid daytime naps!*

After two weeks, Anne noticed that Jim was looking much less tired in the mornings. Jim felt more energetic and less anxious in the second week, and realised that he needed to keep up the changes. Anne also found that her night breathing problems were better, as the evening meal was much lighter and easier to digest. 'Helpful changes for both of us,' Anne shared with Jim.

Self-check on progress

My action plan to sleep well

This is what I will change first or this is what I will do this week:

More information to help support your changes can be found in Resources → : page 354.

Summary of ideas for improving your sleep patterns

Circle ones you tried and found helpful in the circle for helpful sleep patterns.

Helpful Sleep Patterns Circle

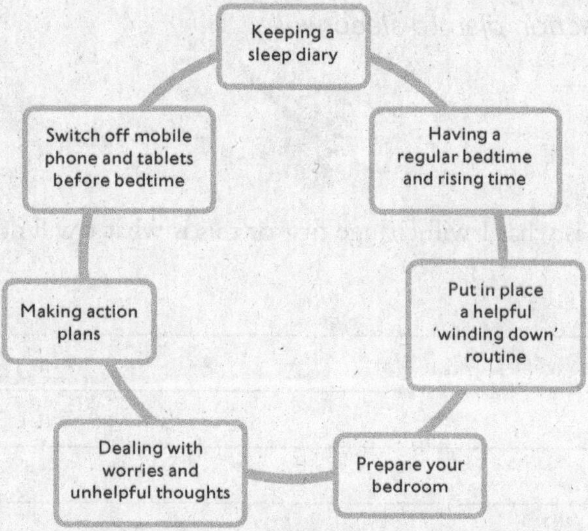

What I learnt in this chapter on sleeping well

- What I found out that was helpful.
- What I tried out.
- What went well when I made changes.
- What got in the way of my changes.
- What next?

Chapter summary

Tick what you valued most in the chapter about managing sleep well.

- ❑ Sleep problems are very commonly reported by people living with chronic pain; both too little and too much sleep.
- ❑ Sleeping well helps the brain and body manage chronic pain better.
- ❑ Sleep patterns *can really* change for the better, so that you feel more energetic, enjoy improved concentration, become more physically active and struggle less with difficult moods.
- ❑ Using a sleep diary can help you to understand your own sleeping pattern. It helps you to be clear about what the problems are, and can guide you to where to start making changes that lead you to sleep well.
- ❑ There are many ways to improve your sleep pattern and prepare for a good night's sleep; pain is managed better as sleep improves.
- ❑ Other things I valued

____

____

____

10

Communication and sharing concerns

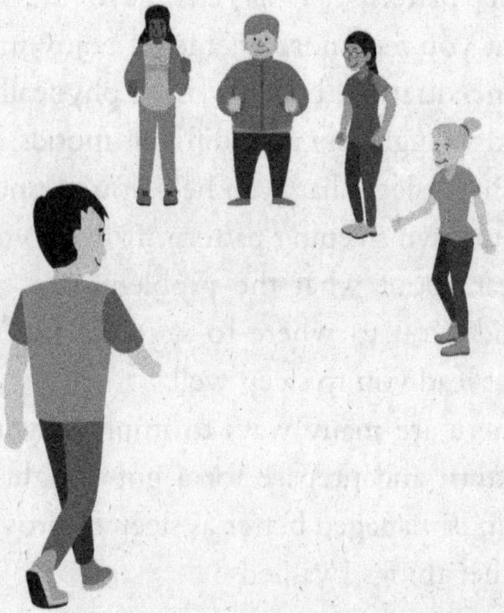

This chapter covers ways of communicating to help close relationships affected by pain. It includes focus on assertiveness and useful ways to talk things through that are difficult and stressful.

Living with pain often means having to speak about it, either to give someone information, to ask for help, or to raise a concern. Sometimes, your partner, family and friends feel closer because they are facing problems together with you. They may know exactly when you need help, when you need to be left alone and when you need to talk.

Sometimes communication becomes more difficult, or even breaks down. It may feel as if their sympathy has run out, or as though they have never really understood how your pain condition affects you. People are different in how much they talk about feelings and what they want. When someone has long-term pain, there may be a fear of hurting feelings, or getting irritable and frustrated.

Explore Jim's story and **underline areas in it** that seem similar to your own.

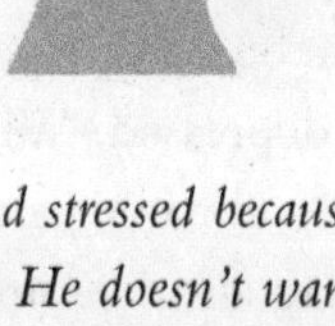

Jim feels irritable and stressed because of the high standards he sets himself. He doesn't want to let Anne know his worries: 'She has enough problems without worrying about me.' They have previously enjoyed an intimate relationship, but due to their health problems this has been 'put on hold', which upsets Anne as it makes her

feel less close to Jim. Anne hasn't talked about this either, as she doesn't want to upset Jim, or make anything worse.

Jim described his situation like this:

'My wife Anne has her own health issues, but she is a very caring person. I am worried that it will upset her if I talk to her about my struggles. I might not be good enough, too. I don't want to put her off from asking me to help her. I know I can get grumpy, too; and I feel really bad when I think I might have hurt her feelings. We have always got on well, and never had any trouble talking with each other, although we didn't really get into deep conversations about things.'

Jim was worried about what Anne might think, but didn't really know because they hadn't talked about it. He ended up feeling a bit stuck and powerless, and wasn't sure how to talk about this.

What can help with communication?

Talking clearly about your feelings and thoughts, and what you need and want, can be hard, especially if you are feeling frustrated, anxious or depressed. Withdrawing from others is a common response to chronic pain and it can help you to cope, sometimes. It may also become an unhelpful habit if it is used too much, and can lead to isolation and loneliness.

Learning to talk about what is helpful to you, saying 'no' and negotiating compromises and solutions, are all very useful skills. And they are needed even more if you are managing chronic pain. At times, it can be very difficult to talk about certain feelings, especially where you have been hurt or painfully abused or suffered trauma. This is where getting support from talking therapists/psychologists can be really helpful in making sense of things, and helping to communicate needs and feelings.

Explore ways to communicate better about pain and your needs

Step 1: Think about your present situation

The questions here explore where communication might be improved.

- Are there times when you feel as if others don't understand what you need?
- Is it difficult to ask for help?
- Is it hard to say 'no' when you want to?
- Do people do too much for you?
- Would it help to be more confident about negotiating or finding ways of compromising with people close to you?
- Does it feel as if people that matter to you have run out of patience with you, or don't care any more?
- Are you withdrawing from social activities?

- Do you feel as if your role at home, at work, or in other settings is taken away or undermined?
- Any there other situations in which you feel your communication isn't working as well as it could?
- Make a note of any situations or meetings that seem relevant to you at the moment. A helpful first step is to be more aware of what is actually happening.

Step 2: Getting ready to talk about it

This next step is to prepare for a conversation.

- Remind yourself about your overall goals in managing your pain →: page 110. If communication is not working very well, then improving it might help you to move towards those goals that are important to you.
- It helps to be clear and specific about what the issues are that need communication. Once you have decided on the issue, you might want to think how to share it and manage your feelings. It may be that you want to raise a concern or ask someone to do problem solving with you.
- Explore management of moods →: from page 237. This is especially if frustration and anger are happening too easily and might get in the way of your communication.
- Choose a good time to have a conversation. Can you find a time when there is less likely to be interruptions, or other extra pressures?

Step 3: Talking about it

Preparation as in step 2 helps you to be clear on the issues that you want to talk about and then to stick with them. Speaking openly in a respectful way helps communication a lot. It means that both partners in the conversation can feel listened to. Where things are tense, or there is a lot of hurt, it can be harder.

It is useful to set the rules for the conversation and to have some key ways to open it; for example, 'I am going to be as open as I can', or 'I need you to listen to me, then I will listen to you', or 'I want to talk to you because I trust/respect/love you'. This can minimise unhelpful interruptions and improve active listening.

> It may help to agree a timed 'listen slot'. This means each person has five minutes to speak, and the other will listen carefully without interrupting. Then the other person does the same for the time agreed. This will help you both to understand what is important to you. You will be able to say what your goals are and the issues that you wish to discuss. Stating how you need to manage your pain better may help them to feel more confident to support and encourage you. It can also help someone not to be over-protective, or not to lose patience with the situation.

You may find that listening respectfully to the other person means that you have more feedback as well. While this is not always comfortable, it means that you know where you stand, and can cooperate to make helpful changes.

You may find it helpful to use the problem-solving ideas ➔ : page 375.

Ways to manage when communication is difficult and stressful

Being assertive can help. Assertiveness is about stating clearly what you want, and what you don't want, while being respectful to the other person at the same time.

Being assertive does not mean getting your own way all the time. Many people worry that if they assert themselves, others will think of their behaviour as aggressive. But there is a difference between being assertive and aggressive.

Assertive people state their opinions, while still being respectful of others. Aggressive people take their own opinions as being more important, and then attack or ignore others. When someone is passive, they don't state their opinion at all, yet may feel frustrated or ignored inside.

The differences between passive, aggressive and assertive ways to communicate

Passive	Aggressive	Assertive
Afraid to speak up or speak at all, speaks quietly.	Interrupts and 'talks over' others, often rushed speaking.	Speaks openly and steadily.
Avoids looking at people.	Glares and stares at others directly.	Makes good eye contact.
Speaks softly.	Speaks loudly or shouts.	Uses an ordinary speaking voice.

What being assertive is like in action with others, family, friends, in the workplace and with healthcare professionals

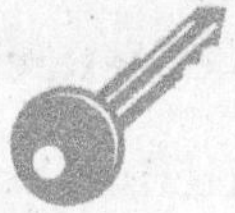

Being assertive includes a number of communication skills. These examples below show ways to be more assertive.

1. **Expressing personal needs or concerns**

   It can be helpful to use 'I' statements about specific needs or worries, like:

   'I want to ask some questions on . . .' or 'I feel scared and worried about . . .'

   'I want to do the washing up myself', 'I would like

you to remind me to do my stretches on . . .' 'I want to talk about how much you do for me . . .'

Or, simply, saying 'No'. . . and then saying 'I feel upset when I say I don't need help and you do it anyway.' Saying 'No' is often quite hard to say to people close to you. Practising saying 'No' and being clear and specific about the reason is helpful. Being prepared and writing down what you would say starting with 'No, and I . . .' usually helps better communication.

With a healthcare professional, it might be, 'I want a longer appointment with more time to talk about the side-effects of my medicines'; 'I want to tell you about my goals'; 'I want us to talk about my self-management plan'.

2. **Avoiding the use of 'attacking' language**

This is often characterised by sentences with 'you' in them. For example, 'You never have time for me'. 'Why did you do this?' Instead, it is more helpful to ask: 'How will the exercises help me?' or 'I feel confused and uncomfortable when I can't get my questions answered'.

3. **Tell the person if the conversation is a struggle**

Share if you feel rushed, or dissatisfied. The only way they can help you is if they know what you are thinking – they are not mind-readers. Let the person know if you need him/her to slow down or you might need to say, 'I can't hear you; please speak louder'.

4. **Ask clearly for information or about concerns**

   So, if the healthcare professional says, 'Don't worry about it,' ask for an explanation assertively, so that you have more information. 'I need to understand more about this, please tell me . . .' For example, you may want to ask, 'I am working on managing myself better, what do you think?' There is more information about ways to talk with your doctor or health care professional in the Resources →: page 377.

5. **Give clear details, and be open about your experience**

   This is especially important with those close to you and healthcare professionals. It may feel easier to say 'I'm fine' or 'I'm not doing so well'. You and others will be able to work together better if you can let them know exactly how your pain is affecting you physically and emotionally. 'I am struggling today as I feel stiffer and slept poorly' or 'I am pretty tired from the medicines so I will do my stretches and relaxation first and then do a shorter walk with you'.

Most of the above are things we might say anyway. If the situation is not going well, or you are unable to agree, there are some techniques that will help.

Explore this example below and circle where Razia is being assertive. Then think about which ones you will try out and practise with them.

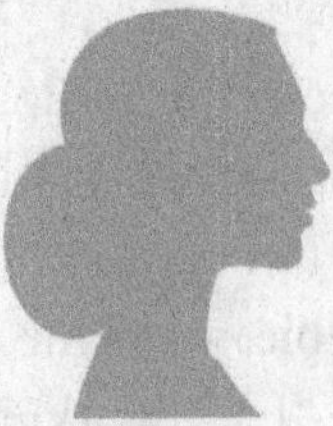

Razia's friend Amaal wanted her to look after Jacob, her five-year-old, for a whole day in the holidays. Razia likes Jacob, and her own children get on well with him. However, at the moment, Razia knows that a whole day would be too much for her, and would upset her pacing plans. She had been practising saying 'no' and sticking to it, in an assertive calm way. The conversation went like this:

Amaal: Razia, please could you take Jacob for the day on Tuesday?

Razia: No. I like Jacob coming over, but I am learning to pace myself, so I can't do that on Tuesday. [Razia has explained herself, but said no.]

Amaal: Please! You know it will help me out, and you have done it before! [Amaal is trying to persuade her.]

Razia: No. I understand your point of view, but I can't do that on Tuesday. [Razia has acknowledged what

Amaal is saying, but has repeated the 'no'. She felt a bit guilty inside, but carried on being assertive.]

Amaal: How about all day Wednesday then?

Razia: No. I can't do a whole day, I am learning to pace myself, so I can't do Wednesday either. [Razia has repeated the 'no' and said the same again – but now she is going to offer a compromise.] If it will help you out, I could do a couple of hours after my husband gets home from work? That would be in the afternoon at about 3 p.m.

Amaal: Well, okay, you know that would help me out. I just need a couple of hours really to get some things done without Jacob under my feet.

In the end, the two friends agreed a compromise that worked for both of them, and that didn't get in the way of Razia's working on her pacing goals.

You can see from this conversation that Razia was polite and respectful, and stayed calm. She repeated what she had to say; and had to keep saying it a few times when Amaal repeatedly tried to persuade her. This is called the 'broken record' skill. It is simply repeating a short sentence that sums up what you want to say, without becoming frustrated.

Explore more →: page 349.

Step 4: Agreeing the next steps

If communication has worked fairly well, you may reach a compromise in which both of you are working together, and understand where the other person is coming from. If things haven't worked well, perhaps it needs more time and thinking space, so that you can try again later. Sometimes if you both agree to forget a previous unhelpful conversation it can help to start again, when ready and more focused and calmer.

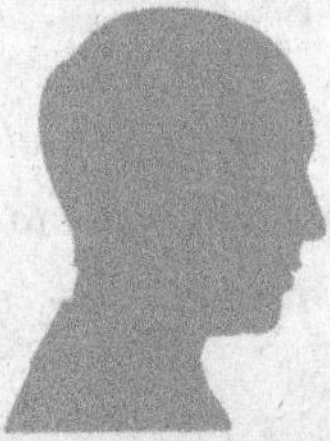

Jim asked Anne if they could have a proper chat over their cup of tea together in the morning. This was a better time of the day, when they were both up and about and not too tired. He was a bit nervous, but he did go ahead. He practised what he would say to start with and promised himself he would listen to Anne without interrupting her. 'I am feeling worried and now very stressed about some things,' he started off, and then told Anne about some of his worries. He didn't tell her everything straightaway. Anne became a bit tearful. He stopped himself from interrupting her. She then explained that she was really relieved he had shared his feelings with her, proceeding to

talk to him more than she had done for a while. They ended up sharing their worries and feeling much closer, with a bit of a plan to deal with some of their worries. Jim felt better in himself, as he understood Anne's thoughts and feelings. He was less stressed too. They decided that talking things through had been helpful and had solved one or two worries. They agreed to have a 'talking date' at least twice a week over a cup of tea.

How to manage communication difficulties in relationships

With practice, you can learn to tell your loved ones what will help you to manage your pain better, and ask them how you can help, too.

For instance, if those around you pay attention to your pain (perhaps by asking, 'How is your neck?'), this can focus your thoughts on it more of the time. In fact, it can make the pain seem worse. People usually *want* to help, and don't want others to suffer. This can sometimes lead to well-meaning concern and being over-protective.

In the long term, all but the most patient people can run out of sympathy or patience with persistent pain. This is when a different approach can help. People close to you need to understand what you are trying to achieve, which is why talking about goals can be useful. Otherwise, they can sometimes jump to the wrong conclusions, which can be unhelpful. It helps to explain clearly how you plan to manage your day or week and your pain.

These suggestions may help those around you to give you the right kind of support. Tick two you might try. If you're not sure, then ask yourself, if your best friend knew your situation, what suggestions they would tick for you.

Tips for improving communication with others to help support your efforts to self-manage of your life and pain.

❑ Share with them information that explains the difference between chronic and acute pain systems in the body.

❑ Ask them to encourage and support you to keep going on your pain management plan.

❑ Ask them to notice when you are trying to cope better, and comment positively.

❑ Remind them *not* to ask you how the pain is (it makes you and them focus attention on it).

❑ Ask them to remind you of your day-to-day success in achieving your goals.

❑ Only offer help when you ask for it, or if agreed it is part of your pain management plan.

❑ Ask then to reward you or do something pleasurable when you are trying.

- ❑ Ask them to do problem solving with you.
- ❑ Let them know that you are not doing further harm by getting active.
- ❑ Accept you are not exaggerating or being lazy as you take rest breaks and 'pace' yourself.
- ❑ Know that you can support, encourage and listen to them in return, even if you are in pain.

How to change patterns in relationships that aren't helping confidence to self-manage

It's well known that if children are rewarded for an action, they are more likely to repeat it. Think about this in relation to yourself. If you are rewarded for doing something, you are also more likely to engage in that behaviour again. Unfortunately, this also applies to unhelpful behaviours as well as helpful ones.

In the short term, being looked after can help; for example, when you have a severe setback. It is less helpful if you are 'looked after' all the time, or others are doing more than they need to. It can make it harder to feel in control of your situation or to believe that you have a useful role to play at home or in life.

Let's take an example of how to change this in helpful ways.

Imagine that you want to get out to the local shop to buy bread and a newspaper. You have chronic pain, which makes you stiff and tired in the morning. Someone who loves you will always offer to do it for you if you tell them that the pain is bad today.

What are the results?

The person goes to get the paper for you, which is kind, but it also means that you are 'rewarded' for saying that you are in pain. The long-term effect on your feelings, pain and behaviour is not always helpful.

Let's imagine a different scene.

You want to get the bread and the paper from the shop every day. You have chronic pain and you are very stiff in the mornings, so it is hard to get started. You set yourself a pacing baseline, planning it so that you can get to the shop if you rest on the bench for two minutes on the way there **and** again on the way back.

Someone who loves you will always offer to do it for you if you say that the pain is bad today.

You explain to them that it would help, instead, to receive a reward, such as a cup of tea, when you get back from the shop. It would also help if they said 'well done' or 'thanks for going to the shop today!' to you, so focusing on your achievements despite the pain and stiffness. You value their support, and ask them to encourage you to go to the shop, especially when you don't feel like it, or are having a bad day.

What are the results?

You still get the paper, while moving towards your goals; and in addition, you are both working better as a team.

As well as this, your partner, family or the people close to you will understand that you are not doing any further harm to yourself by starting to exercise and getting active. They will see that you are not 'slacking' when you slow down, pace yourself, take a break before the job is finished and give yourself a reward for trying.

It is more helpful to be allowed to do things at your own pace, rather than have someone else do them for you. They can then help you with things that you really can't manage, such as heavy lifting.

How to communicate and share your concerns

Talking about living with pain is quite difficult at times. Discussing the questions below with your partner or your family will help towards a shared understanding of how to manage the pain and have better times.

- Do you talk about the hardest part of living with persistent pain?
- What really does help and make it easier to manage the pain?
- And what makes it harder to manage the pain?
- How will you share when you really need help?
- How do you plan to share new goals, new ideas that you would like to try out?

Try out one or two of the suggestions above. Discuss how well the conversation went; try using 'What went well in our talking just then?' and 'What did not go so well and do we know why?'

And remember to reward yourself and your partner and family when your efforts prove successful.

Chapter summary

- It is understandable that communication can be difficult when you have long-term pain. You may need to discuss things that you don't usually speak about; or relationships may become strained when communication isn't working well.
- Learning to talk things over in a respectful way can improve understanding, clear the air, help with problem solving and lead to more progress towards your goals.
- Understanding how to be assertive rather than aggressive or passive can help you to communicate well with people. There are some useful skills and tips that can help clear communication with others.

11

Sexual relations and intimacy

What this chapter covers

Pain and having close physical or sexual relationships can be tricky and at times both physically and emotionally upsetting and painful. If you have a partner, being faced with so many challenges from the pain and life may mean that you need to be close and intimate, perhaps even more than before. Being in pain, or being afraid to cause the other person harm or hurt, can lead partners to avoid physical intimacy. It's important to realise that you can have a physical relationship that works for you as a couple, even when you have a chronic pain condition.

Organisations provide online reading materials, confidential help and advice on sexual and relationship issues →: page 356.

How to improve intimacy and deal with sexual problems

Many people with chronic pain, and their partners, have

sexual problems. Sometimes these begin because of the pain. This can happen when one partner doesn't seem interested in sex, or because the other is fearful of causing more pain or being hurt, for example. Sometimes pain makes existing sexual problems worse.

Dealing with issues makes it more possible to enjoy intimacy, and sex can help maintain closeness and relax both of you. You may find that it reduces stress and relieves pain. Even when you are in pain, your sex drive does not go away, although low mood and anxiety can affect things. Most people still have all their parts in working order, even if they are in pain.

One approach to managing sexual problems is to avoid sex and intimacy. However, this can be upsetting and can add to a couple's problems, especially if they find it difficult to talk things over. Avoiding sexual activity can also lead to avoidance of all physical closeness.

For Jim and Anne, lack of sexual activity was distressing for both of them, especially at a time when Anne needed to feel much closer to Jim. Not talking about it means that sex can become an area of tension, anxiety and may increase pain.

Feelings of failure, frustration and guilt can become reasons for avoiding sexual activity. People often worry about their partner's sexual needs and whether or not having sex is likely to cause problems in the relationship. Many couples have full and contented lives without sexual intercourse. However, if you both want to make changes, it will take understanding, time and commitment to deal with it, rather than avoiding the problem. Both partners need to talk, perhaps several times. It is important to remember that it is a shared problem. Your partner needs to know your thoughts and feelings, so that you both understand exactly what is going on for each other.

For example, your partner may not understand that, even though it is difficult at the moment, you may want to have a sexual relationship in the future.

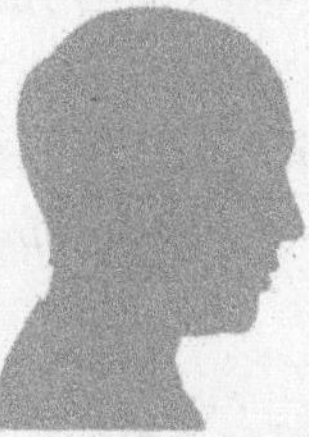

Anne had ended up thinking that Jim was no longer interested in their sex life. She already felt upset about a great many changes in her own health, and she missed being close to Jim physically. He wasn't sure what Anne was thinking, and was a bit embarrassed and nervous about talking about it. After such a long time together, he had assumed that things would 'work themselves out'. At the same time, he hadn't been as physically affectionate towards Anne as usual, because he didn't want to 'put her under pressure'. Trying to talk about the loss of making love seemed a real challenge. After a couple of weeks of 'talking dates', Anne hinted that she would like to speak about their intimate relationship. Jim was also thinking it was time to discuss it. They each shared

their views and feelings, taking time to speak and listen. He began to see what was concerning Anne. They both discovered that the other person missed the physical closeness more than they had realised. They had both wanted to avoid stress and worsening pain, but had ended up losing the togetherness that helped to keep them going. They decided that they would pace themselves by just being close together, touching and hugging more often. Jim would also do some gentle stretches for his legs and back before cuddling Anne in bed. Anne was keen to try this, and was happier that they had a plan in place to work towards a sexual relationship again.

Some ways to make sexual relationships easier and help with intimacy

Pacing

Here are some suggestions for pacing your sexual relationship:

- It's important not to overdo it (either physically or emotionally) to start with.
- Start slowly: set a time together, if it helps you to relax.
- Just try kissing and cuddling, to begin with.
- Both partners need to understand and agree what is

okay at this point. This can help to reduce anxiety and fear about increasing pain (for both partners).

Set some goals together

Set some goals: explore your sexuality together within agreed limits – taking it one step at a time → : page 110.

Full sexual intercourse is not necessarily the long-term goal for everyone. Sexual relationships are more than just intercourse, and there are many alternative ways of being intimate. For instance, many couples find comfort and reassurance lying together, caressing each other, taking a shower together, or massaging each other. Physical satisfaction can be gained from stimulation or masturbating, stroking or kissing. No harm will occur if both partners find this emotionally and physically acceptable.

Practice!!

Some couples find that one or both partners have arousal problems due to lack of practice. Frequent successful practice increases confidence, especially if both partners agree that there will be no pressure to 'perform'.

Pain does not need to be a reason for avoiding a sexual relationship. A couple can become more confident by touching and fondling. With some experimenting and a sense of humour, most couples can work out satisfactory positions that will not cause pain.

Dealing with unhelpful thoughts and feelings

Sex in a loving relationship cannot cause harm to any part of the body. However, like exercising, for the first few times there may be a temporary increase in pain.

Negative or anxious thoughts can make it harder to relax and enjoy sex →: page 242. If you find yourself thinking negative thoughts, you can work together with your partner to challenge them. This will create a more balanced view about being physically closer and sexually active. For example, Jim and Anne shared their concerns. Jim predicted that he would suffer 'awful pain' if Anne touched him around his chest and left shoulder. Jim realised that Anne enjoyed massage with her favourite oils, and that it was pleasurable for both of them. They found that experimenting in this way helped. Jim was less fearful when he realised he did not have to worry about being touched in his sensitive pain areas.

There are pictures of helpful positions for sex in the Appendix →: page 376.

Chapter summary

Sexual relationships and intimacy can improve with a partner. This means communicating sensitively and clearly and working together step by step to overcome obstacles to physical closeness.

12

Managing anxiety, worry and fears

What this chapter covers

In this chapter, we help you to understand more about anxiety and its range of feelings, including worry and fear. We look at what anxiety is and how it can affect people with pain. We then look at what can help in managing anxiety, and how to use these ideas and skills so that you are more able to manage your pain and anxiety well.

Anxiety and chronic pain

People with chronic pain often feel anxious. Pain itself is a threat, and it is normal to find yourself worrying or feeling fearful about many things in life, including changes in yourself and in the pain ➔: page 27.

Below are some of the common worries or fears that people with chronic pain say they worry or fret about:

Pain itself

- How intense or severe the pain is or might become.
- The cause/s of the pain; why I have got it.

Body symptoms and other common issues

- Body symptoms, like numbness or sleep problems.
- Body movements or positions that give severe pain levels.
- Life issues, current and past.
- Staying at work or getting back to work or study.
- Money difficulties, arguments within the family.

How other people perceive or think about them

- Being perceived in critical or negative ways by others.
- Being fearful that people will reject them.
- Being disabled and dependent on other people.
- Being troubled about what clinicians have indicated the future might hold – for example, 'You will need a wheelchair' or something similarly scary or worrying.

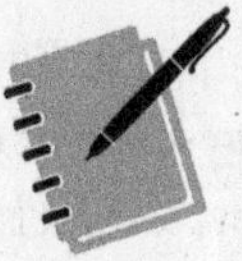

Circle those fears or worries you have. Add any others you have.

____

____

Pain and its Links to the Five Areas

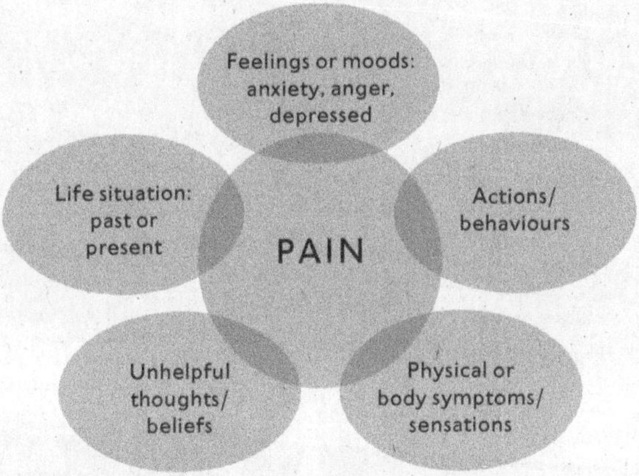

Getting to know more about anxiety

Anxiety can range from physically feeling a bit uneasy or nervous to having a strong sense of dread, emotionally. It can become so bad that the person feels panicky and very frightened. It is normal to feel anxious in some situations. It can help us to stay safe and perform at our best, for example when giving a speech at a wedding, being part of a sporting event, or attending a job or welfare benefits interview. Anxiety is only a problem when it is more severe than you would expect given the situation and when it affects your day-to-day life.

What are the effects of anxiety?

Body Symptoms Linked to Anxiety or Worry

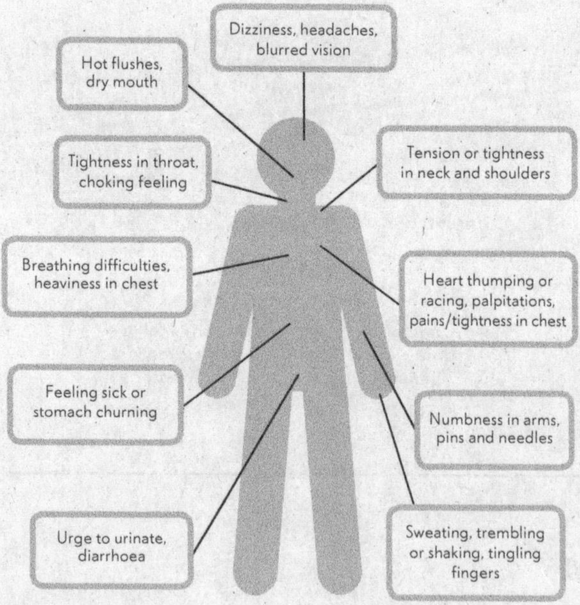

Anxiety affects us in three main ways:

1. Body symptoms and sensations

Anxiety causes the body to react as if there is danger or a threat. It's part of our natural survival system. The body releases adrenaline, a powerful chemical that very quickly makes the heart beat faster and stronger and makes our muscles tense. It gives lots of other sensations like feeling sweaty and shaky, a choking feeling or a tight chest, a dry mouth and dizziness.

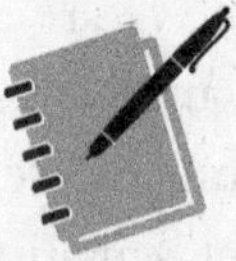

Explore the anxiety and body symptoms diagram and mark your own body symptoms on it.

2. Unhelpful thinking and beliefs

Anxiety and worry can affect what goes through our mind. We might find ourselves making negative predictions and thinking the worst. Sometimes frightening images or pictures can go through our minds, which can turn up the anxiety feelings, increasing the bodily symptoms and sensations. So, the body itself can feel tense, stressed, have tight muscles, gut sensations and so on.

3. Behaviours or actions

When anxious we will stop or avoid certain activities. Anxiety often makes us believe that if we do extra things to keep us safe, the fears or worry will go away. For example, repeatedly checking and feeling a pain area or holding an arm stiffly to prevent any movement that might cause more pain. The result is that the safety behaviours make it even stiffer and more painful!

Ways to manage anxiety: tackling unhelpful thoughts

Anxiety and worry lead to a range of unhelpful changes in the way we think. When we are anxious, we can become fearful about things that might happen and tend to over-exaggerate threats or danger. We feel vulnerable, as our body is full of unpleasant sensations. We believe that we cannot cope and cannot get the help or resources we need to manage the feared problem/s, including more 'horrible' pain. These thoughts make us feel even more worried or frightened, which, in turn, can increase pain.

There are some helpful ways that Jim could use to manage these fearful thoughts and break the negative cycle of fear. We'll take you through them to understand more about how anxious thoughts might be affecting your life and your pain.

Skills and tools to support changes: a Four-Steps-to-Balanced-Thinking approach to challenge unhelpful, fearful or anxious thoughts and achieve balanced thinking

These Four Steps guide you to manage your worries and

fears, and will follow Jim's negative cycle of fear to discover how to use them.

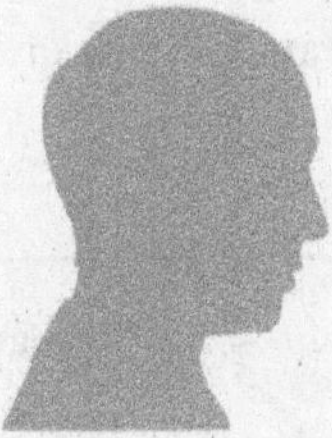

Follow Jim and discover more how he managed his anxious thinking

Jim's story shows how anxious thinking and beliefs feed into a negative cycle that actually makes pain worse.

Jim reached up to put the dishes inside the cupboard. He heard and felt a cracking in his neck. His fearful thoughts instantly took over as he became worried about lots more pain, being out of action and what this would mean for Anne. As his worries increased, his pain increased and so the cycle continued.

Step 1: Start to notice automatic thoughts and feelings

Notice what is actually going through your mind when you start to feel worried or fearful, so begin to have **a Mood Change**. To guide you to notice your thoughts more clearly and build an **Automatic Thought Tracker**, use these questions in each of the columns.

This is Jim's **Automatic Thought Tracker**. As he was feeling more anxious **(a Mood Change)** he began to notice the thinking going through his mind. This is also shown in the negative cycle of fear, see earlier.

Specific situation **What were you doing?** **Where?** **When?** **Who with?**	**Immediate thoughts and negative predictions** **Belief level in these thoughts** **0–100% (where 0 = none and 100% = totally)**	**Feelings, mood** **How bad was the feeling, on a scale of 0–100% (where 100% is the worst possible)?**	**Body symptoms felt**
Jim put the dishes up into the cupboard, when he felt and heard a 'crack' in his neck.	Oh no, the pain will be dreadful for days – I believe it: 80%. I will be stuck here – I won't be able to get to the shops or do anything. I believe it: 75%. No one is here to help care for Anne – I believe it: 90%.	Worried, anxious, scared: 70%. Cross: 60%.	Tight chest; heart pounding; pain: head, neck and arm.

Step 2: Explore the unhelpful thinking styles or errors in the list below and notice any automatic negative thinking patterns.

- Negative or anxious thinking is 'automatic'; that is, these types of thoughts, images or beliefs just pop into our minds very quickly, in an instant!
- They are 'distorted', so when you stop and check them out, they don't fit with all of the facts within the situation or are thinking errors.
- They repeat themselves, sometimes continuously, and as you don't choose to have them they aren't easy to turn off.
- They also seem to be 'true' or 'reasonable' at the time, and unless you stop, challenge and question them regularly, they become familiar and we believe them.

Tick the styles of thinking noticed at a time of feeling anxious.

Tick the styles of thinking you notice with mood changes, e.g. anxiety	Unhelpful thinking styles
Bias against myself	I overlook my strengths. I focus on my weaknesses. I downplay my achievements. I am my own worst critic.
Negative mental filter	I find it difficult to think about positive things. I find it hard to see the positives in a situation.
Fortune telling	I predict the future and expect that things won't go well.
Mind reading	I presume that I know what other people are thinking without looking at the evidence. I often think that others don't like me/ think badly or critically of me. I predict the very worst events will (actually) happen.
Catastrophising	I quickly see small problems or symptoms as a disaster or being very serious, and predict the worst outcome.

Personalisation	I take the blame if things go wrong.
Jumping to conclusions too quickly	I quickly assume the worst when there is no real reason to think this way, and totally believe it at the time.
Bearing all responsibility	I feel responsible for other people having a good time. I take unfair responsibility for things that are not totally my fault.
Making extreme statements/rules	I use words like 'always', 'never' and 'typical' to summarise things. I make a lot of rules that are 'must', 'should', 'ought' or 'got to' thoughts.
Black-and-white thinking	I switch from one extreme to another. I think things or actions are either right or wrong, good or bad.

Jim realised from the unhelpful thinking styles list that he was 'catastrophising', even 'jumping to conclusions', 'using a negative mental filter' and 'fortune telling' . . . Not helpful, so he went on to explore more in the next step.

Step 3: Challenge any negative unhelpful thoughts; discover they may not be 100 per cent true

From the Automatic Thought Tracker, use these **thought challenge questions** below with these negative and unhelpful anxious thoughts:

- Decide how much you believe these thoughts are true.
- Give them a rating from 0 to 100 per cent (0 = not true at all; 100 per cent = totally true).

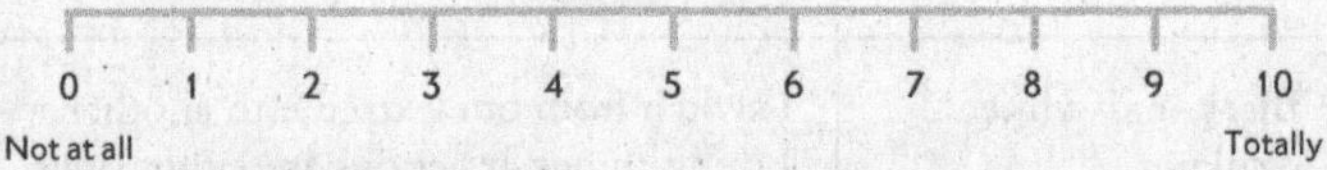

- Write down any evidence that **supports** these negative thoughts.
- Write down any evidence that does **not support** these thoughts 100 per cent.
- Think again about how much you believe the thoughts. Has the rating changed?

Jim's anxious thoughts challenge

*Jim rated these thoughts, **'the pain will dreadful'**, **'I'll be stuck in bed or the house all day'** as 80 per cent true. Then he reflected whether it really made sense to think in this way.*

He checked the evidence.

The evidence ***for*** *his thoughts was:*

- *He heard and felt a cracking sound in his neck.*
- *Anne depends on him to help her do things, like going to the shops.*

The evidence ***against*** *his thoughts was:*

- *I am still able to do things in the house. Even if I have some more pain in my neck, it's not as bad as I predicted. I can pace better now.*
- *Our friend, Jean, can help us if necessary.*
- *I've been in this situation before and I got back on track with the help of my setback plan.*

After reviewing the evidence, Jim decided that maybe his negative unhelpful predictions were not as accurate as he originally thought. His belief in them, that ***'the pain will be dreadful'*** *and so on went down from 80 per cent to 40 per cent.*

Step 4: Develop and practise more balanced thinking

Balanced thinking can lead to being less upset or anxious. This is because you have looked at the evidence about your thoughts/beliefs both **for** and **against** them. This helps a wiser and more realistic range of thoughts to emerge based on facts within a situation or experience. Balanced thinking means you recognise and keep up with all the positive changes that you are making. It helps reduce setbacks and makes you more confident to cope well.

These questions below can help you develop and practise more balanced thoughts and beliefs:

BALANCED THINKING QUESTIONS

- What would your best friend or someone who cares about you say if they knew of these negative thoughts?
- What would you say to them if they had these or similar thoughts?
- Are there any strengths or positives in you or the situation that you are ignoring?

As you become aware of evidence that does **not** always support your negative thoughts, you can practise a more balanced way of thinking and feel less anxious. Over time, this balanced thinking becomes an easier automatic habit.

Coping self-talk skills

A useful skill to help you stay with your balanced thinking when you become anxious is called 'coping self-talk'.

Coping self-talk is what you can say to yourself to remind you that anxiety is an ordinary everyday person's experience, even if it's unpleasant. It can help to write these types of coping self-talk thoughts on a card or in a mobile phone app, so that you have them with you. Try it and see if it helps.

SOME COPING SELF-TALK EXAMPLES ARE:

- Anxiety is normal and can be useful.
- It shows that I'm alert.
- Anxiety is simply my body's response to adrenaline.
- These sensations are not dangerous or serious.
- My body tends to react too strongly to things, as if they are dangerous, when there isn't really a threat.
- It's like a 'false fire alarm'; no fire, just that the alarm went off!
- I've had worries and predicted bad things before, and they didn't happen.
- I can watch the sensations in my body change. They can increase and decrease and go away.
- I can allow the feeling to happen without trying to make it go away, which makes it worse!

Have a go at using the Automatic Thought Tracker and the Four Steps to balanced thinking to guide you to experience less anxiety or worry. If you struggle or find this tricky, then make sure you get more support and help from someone you trust. See Resources ➔: page 369. It may help if you are struggling with trauma or difficult, painful and upsetting life experiences from the past to find professional talking therapy help.

Step 4: Jim developed and practised more balanced thoughts

Jim experimented with a more realistic and ***balanced way of thinking*** *about his situation, using the suggested questions. He came up with:*

- *I am disappointed that I did not do the shopping on my own this week, but at least we have Jean, our neighbour, to help us. I did not spot this positive possibility and I'm grateful for it.*
- *Anne will be fine and understand if I can't do as much as normal; it happens to her too!*
- *I can't be certain that the pain is going to get worse, but, if it does, I have a setback plan to help me to get back on track.*
- *In future, when I have these thoughts, I will tell myself I can only do my best and take one day at a time.*
- *The pain has happened before and went away after a few hours.*

These realistic responses lifted Jim's mood; he felt more cheerful, relaxed and less worried. He planned to watch out for his 'jump to the wrong conclusion' and other unhelpful thinking patterns in future.

He took action and used his setback plan → *: page 331, and was able to get back on track. By actively using his setback plan, it helped his thinking stay realistic and balanced.*

Jim achieved confidence – about 70 per cent in his balanced thinking by using:

- *the Four Steps to manage unhelpful anxious thinking,*
- *and using his setback plan below.*

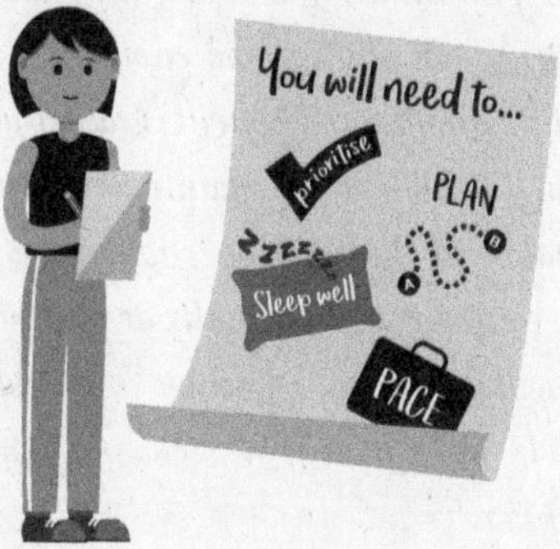

These are some of the things that Jim did that helped:

1. *Stopped cutting the lawn;* ***reduced heavy activities****.*
2. *Did some gentle neck stretches through the day to* ***lessen tense neck muscles****.*
3. *Postponed washing and ironing clothes; still* ***planned to cook*** *supper.*
4. ***Relaxed*** *more; it was sunny and warm, so he sat in the garden.*

His neighbour, Jean, called and offered to take Jim to the shops in her car. This was really helpful, as it meant he could do the shopping, and it also provided a distraction. Overall, Jim's predictions turned out to be exaggerated and unhelpful. He did not experience the severe pain increase he had feared, and he realised he had been more fearful than necessary.

Jim valued the confidence-level rating as a helpful guide to test whether the experiments with the Four Steps to manage unhelpful thinking and setback plan made a difference: 'Seventy per cent is good enough for now; I need to try out this Automatic Thought Tracker and the Four Steps to thought challenging again when I next get anxious. The balanced thinking questions were really good, especially "Are there any strengths or positives in you or the situation that you are ignoring?" It made me realise there was help from Jean if needed and I had forgotten my setback plan.'

THE FOUR STEPS FOR CHALLENGING UNHELPFUL THOUGHTS TO ACHIEVE BALANCED THINKING

Step 1: Start to notice thoughts and feelings; use the Automatic Thought Tracker as your mood changes.

AUTOMATIC THOUGHT TRACKER

Specific situation What were you doing? Where? When? Who with?	Immediate thoughts and negative predictions Belief level in these thoughts 0–100% (where 0 = none and 100% = totally)	Feelings, mood How bad was the feeling, on a scale of 0–100% (where100% is the worst possible)?	Body symptoms felt

Step 2: Identify unhelpful thinking styles (check the thinking styles list above).

Step 3: Challenge your unhelpful thoughts and patterns; discover that they may not be 100 per cent true

- Decide how much you believe these thoughts are true in step 1. Give them a rating from 0 to 100 per cent (0 = not true; 100 per cent totally true).
- Write down any evidence that **supports** these unhelpful negative thoughts.

- Write down any evidence that does **not support** these unhelpful thoughts 100 per cent.

- Think again about how much you believe the automatic thoughts. Has the rating changed?

____

____

____

Step 4: Develop and practise more balanced helpful thoughts

- What would your best friend or someone who cares for you say if they knew of these automatic negative thoughts?

____

____

____

- What would you say to them if they had these or similar unhelpful thoughts?

____

____

____

- Are there any strengths or positives in you or the situation that you are ignoring?

Write your balanced thoughts.

Rate your overall confidence level in this balanced thinking (0 to 100 per cent)

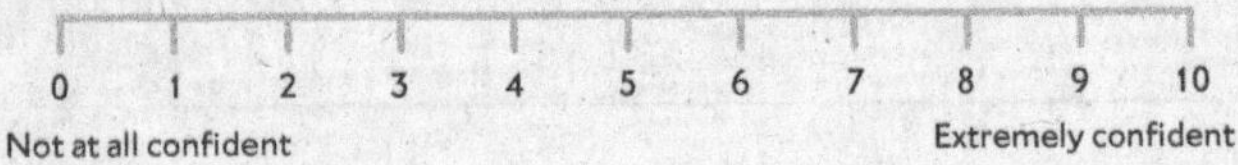

Ways to manage anxiety: staying active and dealing with fears about moving

If we feel anxious, we can do unhelpful things such as change or stop doing activities, or avoid situations that feel difficult. We might not go to certain places, or avoid certain people or activities or times, etc. We may stop doing specific body movements because we worry about the pain or effect they may have on our body.

Unhelpful Cycle of Avoiding Activity to Avoid Pain

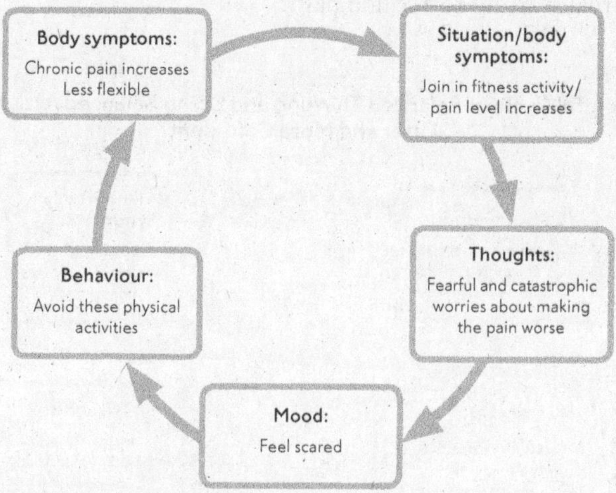

It is common for people with chronic pain to believe that they should avoid movements such as bending, or being more active generally, because they caused pain in the past. In the short term, this seems a sensible strategy. Yet in the long run, it can cause the muscles and joints to become weak, stiff and tighten. This means that bending or other movements are indeed likely to cause pain, as muscles become less flexible; thus the negative prediction seems justified.

A balanced and realistic way of thinking would be to steadily face the feared movements or activities. This would actually stretch the tight, tense muscle groups, help them become more flexible and relaxed, to strengthen the joints and to improve stamina ➔: page 150. This can help to reduce anxiety and increase activity, despite pain. In the long term, it is really likely to reduce pain.

Helpful Cycle of Balanced Thinking and Doing Balanced Activity: Fitter and More Confident

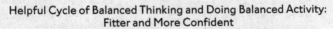

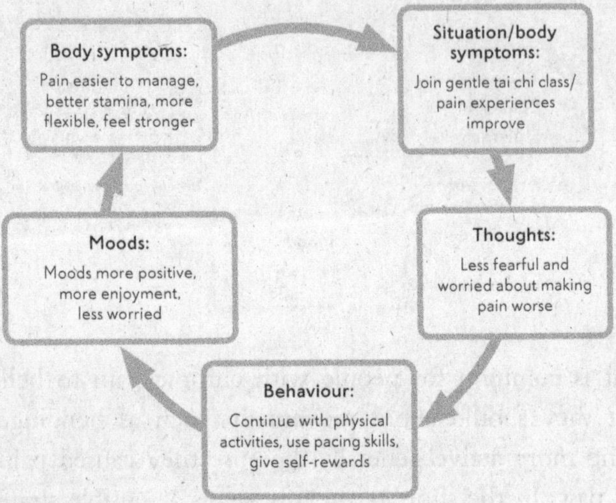

Ways to manage anxiety: using a SMART goal ladder approach

Are there situations where a step-by-step approach might help you to face fears or situations that you avoid because of anxiety and worry? Using the skill of goal setting using Specific, Measurable, Achievable, Realistic and Timed can be helpful to face fears or situations →: page 115.

The goal ladder ➔: page 120 helps guide your planning ahead, prompting you to take small steps to manage your anxieties with more confidence.

Regular practice is the best way to make changes and build confidence. Remember to reward yourself for your efforts, often. Taking too many steps at one time can sometimes cause pain or fatigue setbacks, so remember pacing skills as well.

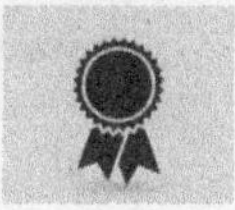

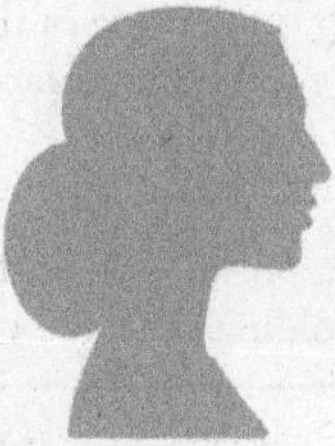

RAZIA'S STEP-BY-STEP TASK:

Razia thought that taking a bath on some days would be relaxing and helpful. She was scared, though, of getting 'stuck' in the bath if she was alone at home, or of making the pain worse, so she decided to use a step by step approach to take this one step at a time to manage her fears. She worked her way through the steps, starting with the least frightening one.

RAZIA'S SMART STEP-BY-STEP GOAL APPROACH

Step number	Task/activity
Start: Least frightening situation:	
1	Sitting on the side of the bath, fully dressed, holding onto the bath rail, feet on the floor.
2	Sitting on the side of the bath, feet on floor, not holding onto the rail at least twice per day.
3	Sitting on the side of the bath, dressed, not holding onto the bath rail.
4	Sitting on the side of the bath, swing one leg in. Practise exercise to help swing legs, especially the hips.
5	Sitting on the side of the bath, swing both legs into the bath.
6	Sitting on the side of the bath, swing both legs and stand in the bath, dressed. Practise sitting-to-standing movements.
7	Sitting on the side of bath, swing both legs and the lower self into the bath with a stool in the bath. Use the grab rails to lift oneself out.

8	Get into the bath filled with water and take a bath while sitting on the stool.
9	Get into and out of a dry bath without the stool.
Most frightening situation: 'Getting out of the bath, falling and hurting myself badly'	

More ways to manage anxiety

Relaxation and unwinding

Learning to let go of tension, practising staying calm and using gentle breathing can all make a difference too. Explore relaxation and reducing tension by learning breathing and relaxation skills →: page 174. Mindfulness skills →: page 42 help us notice thinking, feelings and body sensations **without** becoming involved in them. Using these skills helps the body and mind to be calm and soothed, which helps us manage pain better. The body symptoms of anxiety, especially pounding heart, feeling shaky and others from adrenaline release can be lessened by use of the Out-Breath First skill →: page 277. Explore this valuable quick and effective relaxation skill.

Limit caffeine intake – it releases even more adrenaline

Caffeine stimulates the release of adrenaline, so increases or mimics anxiety symptoms. If you take more than three to four drinks with caffeine in them during twenty-four hours (such as tea, coffee or caffeinated energy boost or soda drinks), this could make your body feel more edgy or anxious. So, check your daily twenty-four-hour caffeine intake and slowly make changes if you need to reduce it. It is important to have plenty of fluids, so try drinking more water. You could also experiment with soothing drinks and foods such as herbal teas, fruit juice or decaffeinated coffee and tea.

Summary of ways to manage anxiety

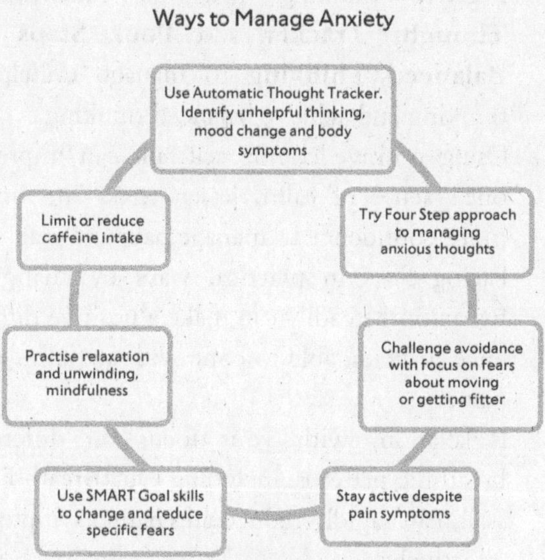
Ways to Manage Anxiety
Use Automatic Thought Tracker. Identify unhelpful thinking, mood change and body symptoms
Try Four Step approach to managing anxious thoughts
Challenge avoidance with focus on fears about moving or getting fitter
Stay active despite pain symptoms
Use SMART Goal skills to change and reduce specific fears
Practise relaxation and unwinding, mindfulness
Limit or reduce caffeine intake

Tick what you found useful about anxiety and managing it.

- ❑ Anxiety, fear and stress are common feelings, and too much of these feelings can make living with pain worse.
- ❑ Understanding more about anxiety and its effects on thinking, beliefs and the body can help the brain and body turn down pain.

- ❑ Using skills to deal with automatic unhelpful negative thinking with an **Automatic Thought Tracker** and **Four Steps to Balanced Thinking** to manage unhelpful thinking and achieve balanced thinking.
- ❑ Using positive coping self-talk can improve one's sense of calm, lessen stress and build more confidence to manage pain and fear.
- ❑ Facing fears in practical ways by changing behaviours steadily can make a positive difference to being able to cope with anxieties and pain.
- ❑ Relaxation, with your focus on different breathing patterns, including Out-Breath First skill, can rapidly reduce adrenaline symptoms effectively.
- ❑ Mindfulness allows the mind to notice anxiety without giving attention to or focus on anxiety, or becoming engaged with the feelings.
- ❑ Other things you valued

____

____

____

13

Ways to manage anger, irritability and frustration

What this chapter covers

This chapter aims to help you understand how anger can affect you and your pain, and other people around you. It explores the links between pain and anger then suggests ways of managing anger and irritability.

Anger, irritability, frustration and chronic pain

Anger, frustration and irritation are very common feelings when you have chronic pain. Everyone has different ways of showing (or hiding) angry feelings. People living with pain can find that they have angry feelings more often, or feel that they become irritated more easily. Someone who used to see themselves as easy-going and tolerant may find that they have a shorter fuse if they experience pain all the time.

Frustrations may lead them to flare up more easily.

Conversely, feeling really irritable and frustrated might cause someone else to 'bottle things up'.

Feelings of frustration, irritability and anger are not always a problem, whether you have pain or not. Some people find that they are happy with the way they express feelings of anger or irritation.

This chapter can help you if you feel that the way you react to angry feelings is unhelpful, and/or is having an impact on the way you manage your pain. Use skills and tools found in the other mood chapters on Managing anxiety, worry and fears →: page 237 and Coping with low mood, depression and loss →: page 290. These include skills of the Automatic Thought Tracker and the Four Steps to manage unhelpful thoughts and achieve helpful balanced thinking' →: page 242.

Useful things to know about anger, irritability, frustration

Usually, we experience feelings of anger and frustration when we fear that there is something (or someone) in the way of what we believe, want or need. So, it may be that we think and feel someone is insulting or attacking us and that they should understand us better. Often things may feel simply unfair, hurtful and unjust, like ending up with chronic pain.

Being in pain can create frustrations if you don't think you can get things done as easily as you used to, to the standard you used to, or be as active. However, there may be other factors triggering your anger, irritability or frustration. You may be dealing with difficulties such as:

- Relationship issues and disagreements.
- Stress at home or at work.
- Not feeling able to meet other people's expectations.
- Money worries.

Drinking too much, and some medicines like opioids or gabapentinoids such as pregabalin or gabapentin, can affect moods. Lack of sleep, tiredness and low energy levels, or being thirsty or hungry or side-effects from medication such as constipation, can add to feeling irritable or edgy.

ACTIVITY: MANAGE ANGER: KNOW YOUR BODY SYMPTOMS OF ANGER EARLY, SO MANAGE EARLIER AND BETTER.

Take a moment to remember a recent anger mood change in the last two weeks where people, events, activities, places affected your mood of anger or irritability or frustration.

As with anxiety, adrenaline is released in the body, e.g. heart starts racing, face goes red, mouth becomes dry, legs feel shaky, etc. Use the body chart found in the Managing anxiety, worry and fears chapter, concerning adrenaline releases the body from → : page 240. Circle the body symptoms you noticed as you became irritable or angry due to adrenaline increases.

Next work with the **Automatic Thought Tracker** to explore the issues about that anger or frustration experience. There is a blank copy →: page 369.

Enter on the Automatic Thought Tracker your body symptoms circled on the body chart in the body symptoms column. Then complete the three remaining columns of the Automatic Thought Tracker using your example of the 'anger' mood change, writing the specific situation or event, the feelings and immediate thoughts and predictions. Follow Maria's frustrated moment to guide you.

AUTOMATIC THOUGHT TRACKER TOOL WITH MARIA'S FRUSTRATED MOMENT

Specific situation **What were you doing?** **Where?** **When?** **Who with?**	**Immediate thoughts and negative predictions** **Belief level in these thoughts: 0–100%** **(where 0 = none and 100% = totally)**	**Feelings, mood** **How bad was the feeling, on a scale of 0–100% (where 100% is the worst possible)?**	**Body symptoms/ sensations**
Speaking on the phone to telephone company for third time at home about a fault in the line.	*Why can't they get this sorted? They should have done it by now.*	*What were you feeling? Very cross.*	***(circled on body chart** →: page 240) dry mouth, trembling legs.*

Exploring the effects of anger on you and your pain

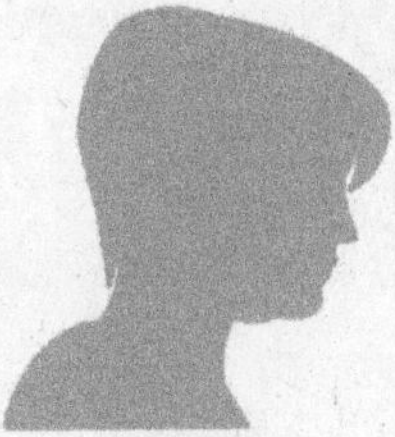

LET'S EXPLORE HOW MARIA'S ANGER AFFECTS HER RELATIONSHIP WITH HER FAMILY

Maria had always been close to all her children, since she had a difficult break-up with their father when they were young. All of them have been trying to support her more since Maria injured herself at work. Maria's daughter, Jeanette, takes her shopping quite often. Recently, Maria lost her cool with a shop assistant and then became even angrier when she could see that Jeanette was embarrassed. They both ended up in tears. Maria was really sorry and said she didn't mean to shout. She was angry with herself for being out of control. Her mood went right down, and she was frightened that she might push her children away.

In chronic pain, you may end up thinking about yourself, other people and the world in a more negative way. There may be good reasons to feel angry about the pain or the events that caused it. It is unfair and it is certainly not your fault. Other people may not understand the pain and the impact it has; they may say or do unhelpful things, often without realising it.

Maria's Anger Experience

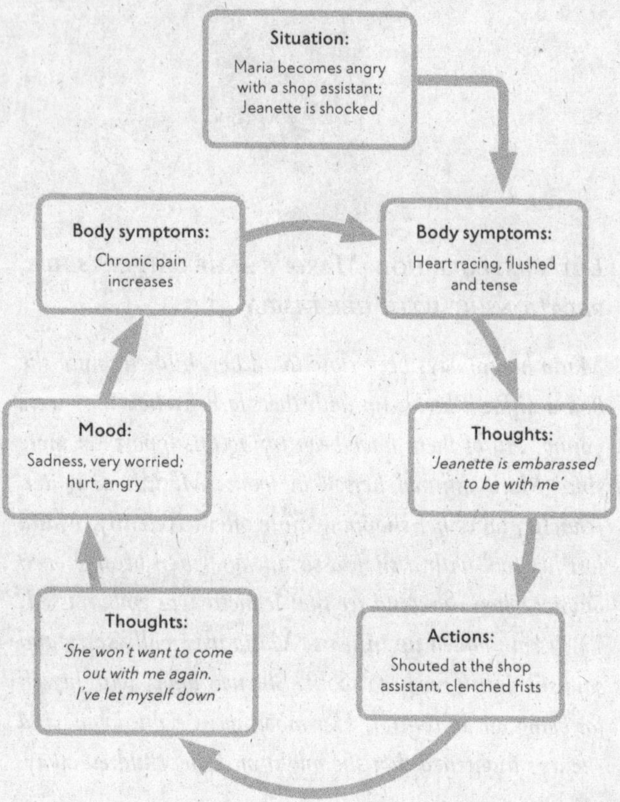
Situation:
Maria becomes angry with a shop assistant; Jeanette is shocked
Body symptoms:
Heart racing, flushed and tense
Thoughts:
'Jeanette is embarassed to be with me'
Actions:
Shouted at the shop assistant, clenched fists
Thoughts:
'She won't want to come out with me again. I've let myself down'
Mood:
Sadness, very worried; hurt, angry
Body symptoms:
Chronic pain increases

While it is understandable to feel angry, if it is expressed in unhelpful ways it can be quite a hurtful experience and makes pain tougher to manage. The brain struggles to manage pain better when there is a lot of anger and fear within the body itself and angry thinking in the mind. So feeling angry and frustrated with negative thoughts can lead to more tension in your muscles and body. This, in turn, can make your body more stiff and tight, thus more pain. Focusing more on the pain leads to a worse sleep pattern, so it is harder to cope with pain. This is an unkind, unhelpful vicious circle, as anger makes pain feel worse and pain in turn make angry feelings worse!!

Like Maria, you might find that your angry feelings are affecting your relationships. People may not understand your situation, especially those you don't know well. Relationships at home may become strained or tense.

Think about the last few times you felt really angry or frustrated and use the **Automatic Thought Tracker** like Maria to record the experience.

AUTOMATIC THOUGHT TRACKER

Specific situation **What were you doing?** **Where?** **When?** **Who with?**	**Immediate thoughts and negative predictions** **Belief level in these thoughts** **0–100% (where 0 = none and 100% = totally)**	**Feelings, mood** **How bad was the feeling, on a scale of 0–100% (where100% is the worst possible)?**	**Body symptoms**

What are the ways I reacted to angry feelings and thoughts?

I said ________________________________

I did ________________________________

Did your anger have an impact on people you care about, or people in other situations? Circle your answer.

YES NO DO NOT KNOW

Looking at the Automatic Thought Tracker, my reactions were:

I said ________________________________

I did ________________________________

Over these pages we explore dealing with anger to see if something else might work better.

Feeling angry is not 'bad' in itself. But how you *react* to your feelings and how you *express* your anger can have an effect on you and your pain.

Let us explore further and start with your Automatic Thought Tracker; if you have not completed this, then try doing so now. An example of how to use the tracker is shown in Maria's case story or ➔ : Jim's on page 244.

Ways to manage anger, irritability and frustration

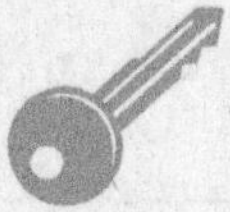

Here are some helpful ideas for managing your anger and frustration.

Explore them and use your Automatic Thought Tracker record and choose one or two of the suggestions below to experiment with managing your thinking, reactions or your body sensations.

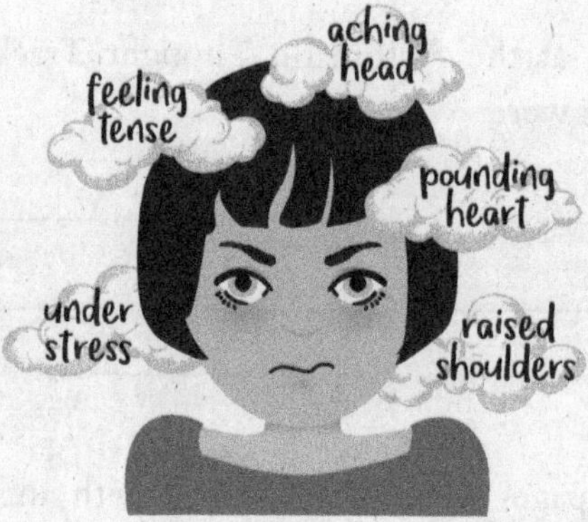

1. Coping with the adrenaline rush in the body

Body feelings of anger are a totally normal reaction to a stressful experience. The adrenaline that is released into your system makes your heart beat faster, your body tenses up, and you may get flushed or sweaty – this is sometimes called arousal. These bodily feelings are all part of your body's natural 'fight or flight' survival response. Our bodies are not designed to be in a state of arousal for a long time and usually such symptoms will calm down after a short period.

If the angry feelings and sensations continue to rise . . . practise taking a pause – try not to respond immediately and try . . .

Out-Breath First skill, which rapidly helps your body to become less tense and reduces the effects of the initial adrenaline rush, winding you down. In anger as tension in the body rises, it seems natural to take a big IN-breath and then OUT-breath. It is really more helpful as the anger body symptoms and thoughts emerge to focus on the OUT-breath first, as if emptying out all the air from the chest through your mouth. This 'blow away the anger' gives your body and mind a signal to unwind and reduce tension. Then settle into a pattern of breathing where your out-breaths through your mouth are longer than your in-breaths through your nose. **Count the out-breath to four or longer up to seven and only count three for an in-breath.** It is helpful to practise this when you are calm so that you are really set for challenging situations and pain. Use this skill for around four minutes or more as this pattern of breaths helps letting go anger and tension and breathing in relaxation and peace helps block the adrenaline effect on the body. It also slows down over-reactive, sensitive thinking too.

2. Managing angry thinking using your Automatic Thought Tracker record of an anger mood change with its angry thoughts

One way is to use some helpful self-talk questions and their answers like these below:

- What is making me angry now?
- Have I listened properly?
- Have I got all the facts about this event or situation right?
- Have I got the whole story?

It will help you to think more slowly and calmly, taking time to think about what will happen afterwards if you react differently.

More useful things to ask yourself when the situation has become 'hot' and angrier:

- Have I been clear about what I want – maybe not?
- Have I jumped quickly to conclusions or made a mistake?
- Are there any other ways to explain the situation?
- Am I really choosing the conflicts that I want to fight right now?
- Is it worth getting angry about this now?
- What will the 'fall-out' be for me or others?

3. Taking time out skill to manage anger mood changes

Ask for 'time out' in the situation for:

- space to think before responding;
- getting the facts clear;
- the opportunity to check through ways to express your feelings helpfully.

In 'the space to think', explore the self-talk questions on the previous page and their answers, along with your Automatic Thought Tracker skill with Steps 2 to 4 in the Four Steps, to manage and achieve balanced thinking →: page 370.

For example:

- What would your best friend or someone who cares about you say if they knew of these angry, negative thoughts?

Summary so far of some useful ways of dealing with anger.

Telling yourself that you are strong enough not to let this wind you up may be helpful. Listening more, or simply waiting a bit longer, perhaps using Out-Breath First breathing or other relaxation skills can allow calm down time for you to see the bigger picture, a different perspective or a new solution. Using the Automatic Thought Tracker questions as soon as you are aware of emotions rising can help redirect your thoughts to looking at alternative explanations.

4. Types of self-talk to use when you still feel wound up

If you are dealing with conflict or being wound up by others, try these self-talk ideas, and if they prove helpful, jot down in a notebook or on a mobile phone the useful ones for the situation and in the future.

Tick the self-talk ideas you want to try.

- As long as I keep my cool, I'll be in control of the situation.
- I don't need to prove myself now or here.
- STOP – there is no point in getting mad or cross.
- Look for positives, watch out, don't jump to conclusions or catastrophise.
- Let's take the issue steadily and slowly, point by point.

- I will deal with it in helpful ways even if they want to make me angry!
- My own self-talk ideas . . .

____

____

____

5. Preparing for a situation that you know can get you angry

Sometimes you will know in advance that a situation or person is likely to wind you up. This gives you some time to prepare, and thus options to deal with it steadily, without anger feelings interfering and with fewer effects of adrenaline on the body and more pain.

If it feels personal, practise not taking it personally. Stick with the issue only and see if this helps with better managing how you express your feelings and your pain.

Use a plan to manage feelings of anger and adrenaline arousal as they occur, such as consciously relaxing the body areas that get tight as you get angry or frustrated, and using the Out-Breath First skill routine above.

Maria found it was her neck and shoulder that became tight and she purposely relaxed them as she felt the tension build.

Use time outs to give yourself space for thinking through the conflict issues.

6. Communicate feelings of anger in a helpful way

Here are some tips on finding other effective ways of communicating about your angry feelings:

> MORE SELF-TALK IDEAS
>
> - Stop for a moment, check what the issue really is, and focus on that only.
> - Share how you feel, avoid 'blaming' someone else, stick with the issue itself.
> - Suggest how someone can change their behaviour if it is making things difficult for you. Do this in a respectful way.
> - Watch out for 'black-and-white thinking'. It can help to move away from seeing yourself or the situation as *totally* right or wrong.
> - Give time and attention to understand the other person's point of view; 'get inside their shoes': it is often a very different view!
> - Stop plotting revenge – it needlessly saps the mind of energy, and it is not worth it, ever.

After the event, the angry or frustrated mood experience

If you have felt really angry or frustrated, this can be an opportunity to check with yourself whether you dealt with things in the way you hoped. Then, if needed, you can adjust your coping plan, or do some more practice on ways to manage anger.

It may be useful to look at problem solving →: page 327 if the situation has remained unresolved. You can always do some relaxation and return to it later. If you feel you did well, remember to tell yourself that you handled it well, even if the issue isn't resolved. Make a note of what you've tried, and keep a log of what you are managing better despite the pain. You can use your Positive Diary Log to do this. These skills are your own collection of evidence that you are managing life better despite the pain →: page 324. Rewards also help reinforce helpful things that work well.

If you're not happy with how it went, remind yourself that you are experimenting. It is just another experience to learn from. Then decide what you would prefer to do and **not** do next time.

If the situation is resolved, remember to tell yourself that you dealt with it well and didn't allow yourself to get too wound up by it. You may think, 'I am getting better at this all the time'; or, 'I could have got more upset, but it really wasn't worth the aggravation', or even, 'I know they didn't mean to be that insensitive, and I can be the bigger person here'. It helps to be both kind and supportive in your thinking about yourself and your attempts. Being self-critical makes your anger and anxiety systems over-sensitive and over-reactive and unhelpful for dealing with pain.

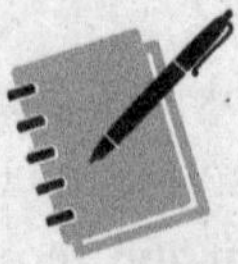

USING THESE SKILLS TO MAKE YOUR OWN ANGER COPING PLAN

This will guide you in what to do if you begin to feel attacked, frustrated and angry. Remember to include:

- ways to handle increased tension and adrenaline-driven body sensations as the angry feelings set in;
- questions to check angry and frustrated thoughts going through your mind.

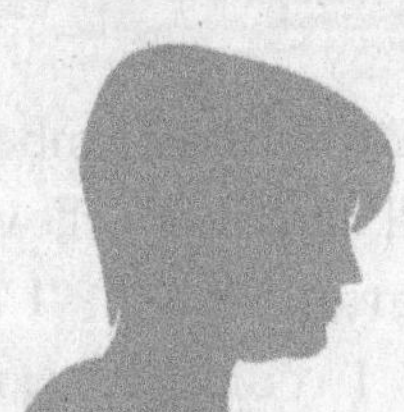

Look at the notes above and Maria's plan below to guide you in creating your own plan. Here is an example of how Maria used her plan to manage anger in a specific situation.

Maria's Anger Coping Plan WAS based on these suggestions

1. **Choosing when to talk:** She talked over her angry

feelings with her daughter, Jeanette, when they were both calmer. Jeanette helped Maria with her plan.

2. Practise self-calming: To start with, Maria practised calming herself down physically, by practising the Out-Breath First skill →: page 277 when she wasn't angry. This meant she would be more able to use breathing techniques in difficult situations or as angry feelings started up.

3. Making setback plans: Maria noticed that her temper was worse when the pain was severe. She made a plan for coping with pain setbacks. Having this plan gave her more confidence to deal with such difficult times, and she felt less frustrated.

4. Checking for balanced thinking: Maria started taking a step back, and checking her thinking, by saying to herself, 'So what is *really* the issue here?' She challenged thoughts that didn't help, by thinking of other possible explanations for them, i.e. using the self-talk questions, see above. She found it easier to spot her unhelpful thinking styles of 'jumping to conclusions' and 'black-and-white thinking'.

She used her 'best friend question' a lot to get a balanced view →: page 250.

5. Shifting focus on practical helpful actions: She became less wound up about standing in queues thinking about how unbearable her pain was. She chose this time to calm her breathing, and focused more on what to say to the assistant at her turn. She was interested to find that if she remembered to pause and smile, she received more friendly responses. This helped her feel successful and less frustrated as well.

RESULT: Maria began to handle events more calmly and was less irritable.

Maria goes shopping with her daughter Jeanette, usually on a Wednesday. Sometimes Jeanette arrives late, which means that Maria has to rush her shopping. This makes her tense because she is worrying about when Jeanette will arrive. She knows that if she rushes round the shops, she gets more pain. If she is short of time, she is more likely to start getting wound up if she has to wait in a queue. She is more likely to start feeling irritated, and have thoughts like 'I wish I didn't have to rely on Jeanette, I used to do all this myself', 'I wish I could do it on my own'.

MARIA'S PLAN FOR MANAGING ANGER WHEN SHOPPING

- *I will explain to Jeanette why I get wound up, and check whether we can solve this together. I haven't told her before, and she can't read my mind.*
- *I'll tell myself there is no need to get cross. I am grateful she helps me, even though I wish I didn't need to rely on her.*
- *Maybe I'll suggest we go at a different time when she isn't rushing; that might be better for both of us.*

- *I'll prioritise if we are short of time, so that we focus on the most important thing to get done.*
- *I'll use the breathing exercise if I start to get tense.*

Maria realised it was helpful to talk through important issues at a time when both she and Jeanette were calmer. She found that they were both then more able to focus, and get more done, by taking breaks and not trying to do everything all at once.

Maria also started to watch for ***body symptoms*** *as she became frustrated, in order to 'nip them in the bud'. She noticed her temper flared up if she was more tired, so this was a good time to practise slowing down and the Out-Breath First skill. She shared with Jeanette when she was becoming tired, and suggested more breaks.*

Plan your own Anger Coping Plan; choose two or three ideas and create one here.

If a plan does not work the first time, then look to make changes or experiment with it. Try at least three times to work out if it is the best of plans!

Summary of ways to manage anger and frustration

Tick below the ways to manage anger that you will try out.

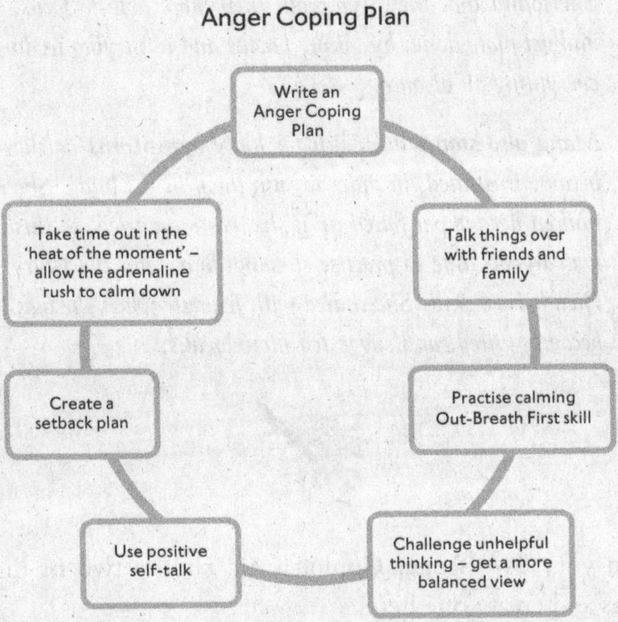
Anger Coping Plan
Write an Anger Coping Plan
Talk things over with friends and family
Practise calming Out-Breath First skill
Challenge unhelpful thinking – get a more balanced view
Use positive self-talk
Create a setback plan
Take time out in the 'heat of the moment' – allow the adrenaline rush to calm down

Summary of dealing with anger and frustration

- Feelings of anger, frustration and irritation are common emotions, and are usually connected to feelings of being blocked, treated unfairly, or attacked.

- Anger affects feelings, thoughts, behaviours and body sensations, and can affect the experience of persistent pain.
- It is possible to express anger in a 'healthy' valued way. Responding to situations calmly, even if we are angry and frustrated, will make it easier to manage ongoing pain. This can be done by learning different ways to deal with unhelpful thoughts, feelings and body sensations.
- Using and changing Anger Coping Plans can help to deal with situations that make you angry.
- Building these skills, especially the Out-Breath First skill, to manage anger well helps build a 'kinder and confident' self and lets pain take a back seat.
- Rewards help to build up confidence in skills you tried out and found useful.

14

Coping with low mood, depression and loss

What this chapter covers

In this chapter, we explore feelings of low mood, including depression and grief, and how we respond to losses in life. We learn more about how and why people get depressed and how it affects thoughts and actions. Then we focus on what skills you can use to help deal with low moods yourself when life and pain are difficult. There are suggestions about resources you can use, and where you can go for extra support.

Low mood, depression and loss, and chronic pain

Chronic pain is stressful and can contribute to feelings of unfairness, helplessness and frustration. It can cause tiredness because sleep patterns are interrupted. Pain is likely to bring changes and losses, such as with work or friends or of self, 'loss of the person I used to be' and at times feel less meaning in life itself. It can also mean less enjoyable activity and less time with others. It is understandable that people with chronic pain struggle with low moods. Other factors including side-effects from medicines for pain relief (such as strong opioids) can cause low moods or mood changes.

If you have chronic pain and low mood, you may find that it can turn into a negative 'chain reaction'. Feelings of frustration, loss and anger can lead to low mood. Having low moods means negative thoughts are exaggerated with unhelpful thinking styles, so viewing the future as more hopeless. This negative thinking then keeps the depressed and sad feelings going. These negative thinking changes are not a 'person's fault'; they happen and are due to depression, which is an illness.

Low Mood Cycle

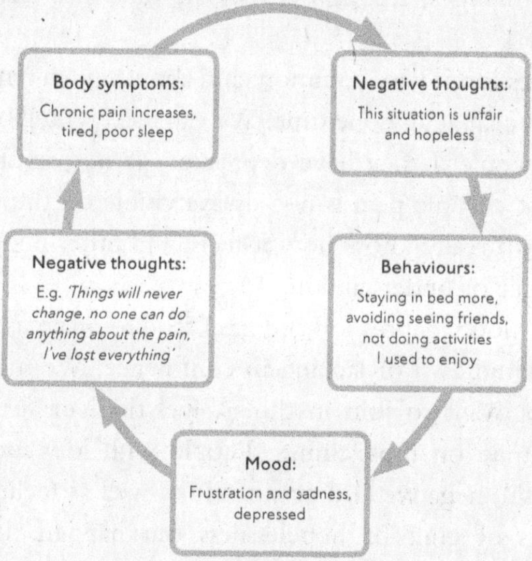

How and why do people have low mood and depression?

Feeling sad and low are ordinary feelings that we get when we have losses in life or when something bad has happened. It's normal to grieve over losses, even if the sadness lasts for weeks or months. People who are grieving usually stay connected with their day-to-day life, and gradually function better as they get used to their loss. However, when sadness and low mood affect our mental well-being for most of the day, every day, and when we lose a sense of hope, or there is no enjoyment at all, then we call it depression. In depression, there are many body symptoms too like sleep difficulties, feeling tired all the time and changes in appetite.

Depression is very common, and about one in ten people experience it at any one time. We can't always tell by looking at people if they have depression or not, in the same way that chronic pain is not always visible on the outside. Only **you** really know how it feels, and other people may not notice or understand it.

Low mood, depression and grief tend to make us quieter, more withdrawn or lacking in confidence. We may laugh less, not want to join in things, feel tired or struggle to concentrate on most things. People with low mood can be tearful, negative and pessimistic as well as feeling tired. Feelings of guilt or hopelessness can happen. It affects relationships because of a general lack of interest or energy, as well as being less interested in sex or intimacy. Sometimes people use alcohol or smoke cigarettes or vape far more. Often they use drugs – like opioids, such as heroin, or other drugs, such as cannabis or cocaine – to help them forget or soothe sad, traumatic or hurtful times or experiences for a short time. In the longer term, this can add to their difficulties. Others hide the way they feel by laughing, smiling and joking around. Feeling low and depressed really does have many faces.

Some of the medicines that you take to reduce pain may add to your feeling low or depressed. Many people who have used strong opioids like morphine or oxycodone find they cause depressed moods, which lessen when stopped.

→: page 377

If you are uncertain whether you are depressed, ask yourself about the last two weeks: how often, over the time, have you been bothered by any of the following problems?

1. Little interest or pleasure in doing things.
2. Feeling down, sad, depressed or hopeless.

If the answer to the two questions is yes and both of these problems are happening nearly every day or more than half of the days, then you may be depressed. If you are struggling to manage it, then it is time to ask for extra help. This is sometimes not easy, yet there is really good help and support available from trusted people like your family doctor and/or professional mental healthcare services. This can really make a difference, and many people who struggled with depression and got help were pleased they did so. 'It is an illness and needs supportive and kind treatments to help change the depressed feelings and thinking.'

It may help to share with them your notes, or examples of a depressed mood, or even your Five-Areas tool →: page 363 and Resources →: page 349.

If you are struggling with side-effects of prescribed medications such as strong opioids, then seek professional help to reduce and stop safely without withdrawal symptoms. Help is also there if you want to change or stop any other medication use: alcohol, cannabis or heroin, for example.

We have used the Five-Areas tool →: page 9 to explore the impact of pain. We can use this same model to understand feelings of low mood/depression. Let's have a look at how the 'Five Areas' can help us understand Razia's depressed feelings.

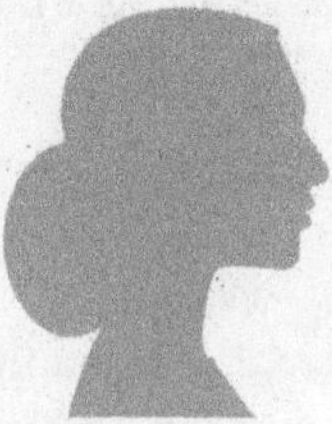

Razia has realised that she has some depressed feelings. Her mood had been very low for a few months after the birth of Ali, her second child, five years ago. Now she is having some of the same feelings and experiences again. She worries about her fibromyalgia pains and what it might mean for her and her family in the future. She is frustrated that 'I can't do the same things that I used to, like cooking, which I enjoy, walking to the park, visiting family and friends.' The way that the pain varies day to day for no reason makes it feel even more out of control.

She feels very stiff in the mornings, and finds it hard to get going, just at the time when she has to manage getting the children ready for school on her own. She generally feels she's 'just not good enough'. This is how she believes Hassan's parents see her too. She feels 'defeated'; as if she 'can't win and it is a bit hopeless'.

When Razia used the Five-Areas tool to look at her situation, it helped her to make sense of why she was feeling depressed.

Razia's Life Situation Using the Five-Areas Tool

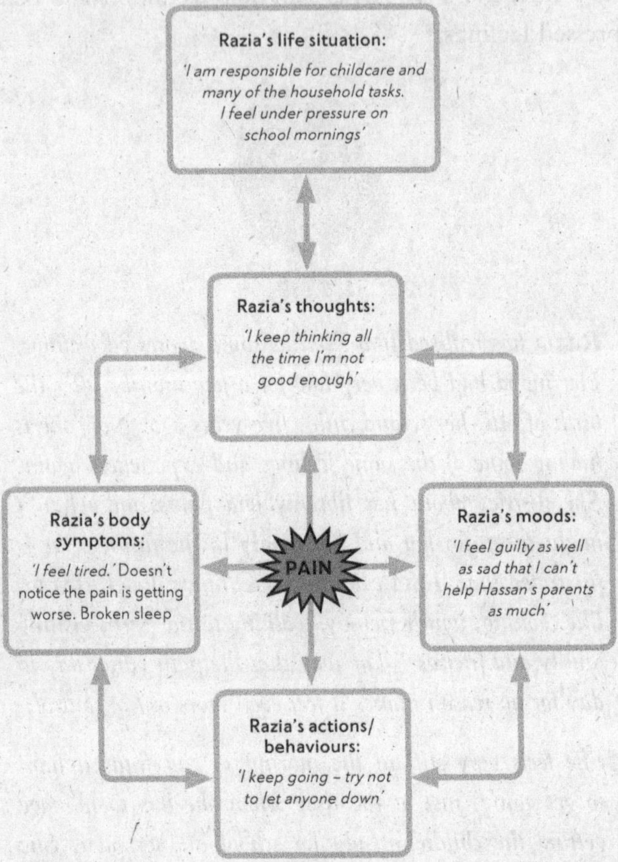

Razia's life situation:
'I am responsible for childcare and many of the household tasks. I feel under pressure on school mornings'
Razia's thoughts:
'I keep thinking all the time I'm not good enough'
Razia's body symptoms:
'I feel tired.' Doesn't notice the pain is getting worse. Broken sleep
PAIN
Razia's moods:
'I feel guilty as well as sad that I can't help Hassan's parents as much'
Razia's actions/ behaviours:
'I keep going – try not to let anyone down'

Make a note of any factors that you think may be linked to your own depressed mood at present, using the Five Areas of the person:

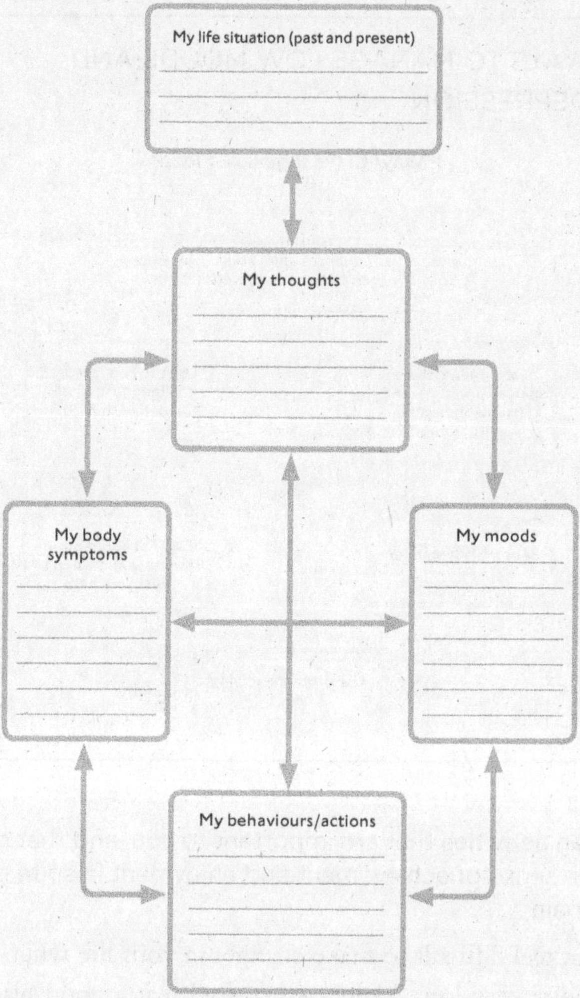

Ways to manage low mood, depression, grief and loss

There are a number of things you can do to help with your low mood.

WAYS TO MANAGE LOW MOODS AND DEPRESSION

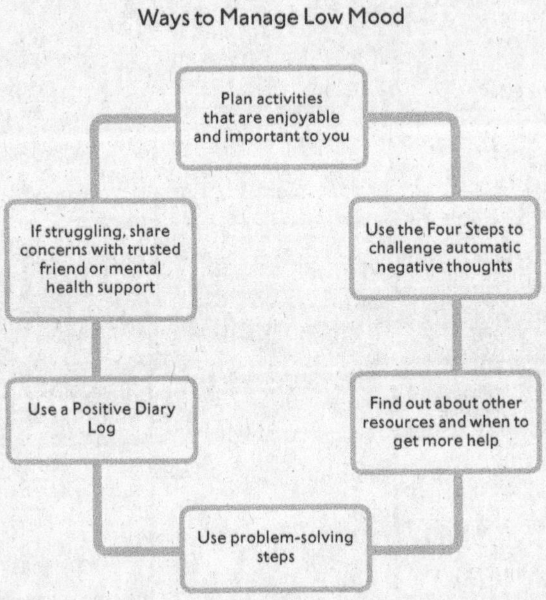
Ways to Manage Low Mood
Plan activities that are enjoyable and important to you
Use the Four Steps to challenge automatic negative thoughts
Find out about other resources and when to get more help
Use problem-solving steps
Use a Positive Diary Log
If struggling, share concerns with trusted friend or mental health support

1. Plan activities that are important to you, and that give you a sense of achievement and enjoyment in spite of the pain

It can feel difficult to make changes in your life when your mood is very low. Many people find that a good place to start is to focus on the things that really are most important to you. For Razia that is the care of Ali and Yousef, ensuring that they enjoy home and school life. This type of focus helps with getting motivated and spending energy and effort on what is really valuable and also brings a sense of enjoyment.

To help with low or depressed moods, explore doing things you might find rewarding or enjoyable. They can help you to keep going when it's hard. It helps to be kind and supportive to yourself, as you also have pain to deal with. Pacing and balancing activities, along with giving yourself rewards, all help the mind to become more aware of pleasant happier moods and to be less depressed. If stuck for ideas concerning enjoyable activities, there are suggestions at the back of the book →: page 352 and 379.

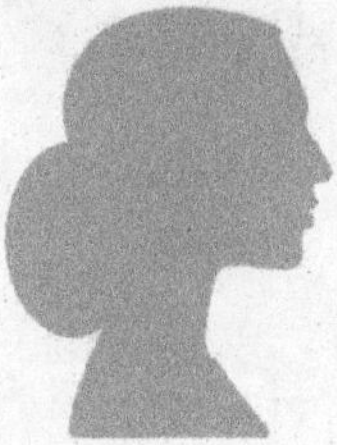

Razia found spending thirty minutes in the park after school with Ali and Yousef lifted her moods. She liked hearing them laugh, and playing with them meant she felt brighter and like a 'proper mother'. She rewarded herself and them too with an ice cream in the park café. She decided to do this activity twice a week, even if she had a setback. Planning

and doing it motivated her, and she would just pace it with care if her pain flared up.

Making small changes to one of the Five Areas can have a positive effect on the others →: page 11. For example, if sleep is a problem, planning changes to your sleep routine to improve it may make you feel more energetic (**body symptom**) and more enthusiastic (**mood**). You may be able to do a few more activities at home with family or friends (**actions**). You might then think: 'I am feeling a bit better because I can do this and the family are supportive' (**more realistic positive thinking**).

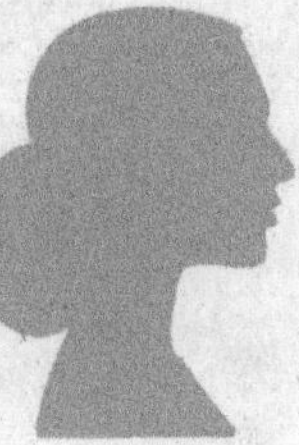

RAZIA'S ACTIVITY PLANS

For Razia, it was helpful to write down all the things that were affecting her mood. She could see why she felt sad and that it was time to be kinder to herself. She decided it might help to talk it over with Hassan. It did help, and they both started on a plan of action by making a timetable of ***all the activities*** *to be done each day in the week. They checked how this was looking at the* *moment, and then started to plan for the next week; Razia made sure the plan included within it the most important and necessary things to be done.*

They focused on activities that Razia thought were most important to her, particularly how she cares for the children and Hassan's parents.

Monday's plan looked like that shown below. Tuesday to Friday were exactly the same.

ACTIVITY PLAN; WHAT HAPPENS NOW FOR RAZIA USING HER ACTIVITY PLAN TOOL AS SHE RECORDS HER ACTIVITIES

Activity Plan	How to use an Activity Plan Track your activities through the day and night. Write them down and rate how much: • satisfaction or sense of achievement, with the scale range A = 0, no achievement, and 5 = maximum achievement; • enjoyment or pleasure, with the scale range P = 0, no pleasure at all, and 5 = extremely pleasurable, e.g. walked in the park: 2/5.
Time of day or night	Monday
a.m.	Get up at 6 a.m. to take tablets. 6.30 a.m. – quick wash and get dressed: A = 2/5. Wake children. Start preparing breakfast, do packed lunches: A = 3/5.

	Get the washing on: A = 2/5. Help children get dressed, find their school bags, etc.: A = 3/5, P = 2/5. Get their shoes and coats. Walk to school with children: P = 3/5. Walk back and get a few items from the corner shop: A = 3/5. Call in on Hassan's parents: P = 3/5. Put their washing on, do some tidying and have a cuppa with them, check if they need anything for later: A = 4/5. Go home.
p.m.	Resting – too much pain: A = 0/5. Start to prepare evening meal. Collect children. Walk back talking about their day: P = 4/5. Finish preparing evening meal: A = 3/5. Help children with homework: P = 2/5; A = 4/5.
evening	Have evening meal as a family. Do the washing and cleaning up. Children's bedtime routine. Watch TV with Hassan for thirty minutes: P = 4/5.
night	Bed 9 p.m. to 6 a.m. Slept some of the time.

Razia noticed from the timetable that she was trying to fit everything in early in the day, before she was in too much pain or very tired. She realised from exploring the pacing chapter that she was in a 'boom or bust' activity cycle. She saw she was probably overdoing jobs, felt more tired and this made her feel low. She and Hassan used the Five Steps Problem Solving tool → *: page 375. They realised the problem was that Razia was getting stuck in the 'must do everything today' thinking trap. Razia decided to focus on the real priorities in the morning, and, with Hassan, she agreed on small changes to her morning routine. For example, she would take a short rest with relaxation after taking the children to school and not check every day if Hassan's parents needed anything.*

This planned change in her routine was to be an experiment. The experiment was to see whether, if she made a change by taking a relaxation break, undertook an enjoyable activity and made fewer checks on her parents-in-law, she would then feel less tired, brighter and more optimistic. So what really happened?

The problem for Razia was the feeling that she is 'letting Hassan's parents down', which made her feel guilty and a bit more depressed → *: page 296.*

Razia had discovered she could spot her 'negative mental filter thinking' and her unhelpful thinking styles. She had learnt about these in ways to manage anxiety and automatic unhelpful negative thinking → *: page 242.*

She also realised she had ignored the fact that Hassan's brother visited his parents twice a week, so she could safely visit less.

Their new plan now looked like this, and so Razia felt more confident.

RAZIA'S NEW ACTIVITY PLAN

Razia's new activity timetable here shows the activities she planned from Monday to Friday (Only Monday is given here, as an example.)

Activity Plan	How to use your Activity Plan Track your activities through the day and night. Write them down and rate how much: • satisfaction or sense of achievement, with the scale range A = 0, no achievement, and 5 = maximum achievement; • enjoyment or pleasure, with the scale range P = 0, no pleasure at all, and 5 = extremely pleasurable, e.g. walked in the park: 2/5.
Day- or night-time	Monday
a.m.	Get up 6 a.m. to take tablets. 6.30 a.m. – quick wash and get dressed: A = 3/5. Wake children. Start preparing breakfast. Help children to get themselves dressed and their school bags ready, etc.: P = 2/5; A = 3/5. Let them get their shoes and coats. Walk to school with Ali/Yousef: P = 4/5. Walk back and get a few items from the corner shop. Go home and have a rest for thirty minutes, either reading or listening to my favourite music, or doing my relaxation: P = 4/5.
p.m.	Start to prepare the evening meal (I can sometimes cook double and freeze some for a day when the pain is more difficult to manage): A = 3/5. Visit Hassan's parents for a cuppa on the way

	to the school to collect the children: P = 3/5; A = 3/5. Collect children: A = 3/5. Walk back, talking about their day: P = 4/5. Get the washing on: A = 3/5. Finish preparing the evening meal: A = 3/5. Hassan and I both help the children with homework: P = 4/5; A = 4/5.
evening	Have evening meal as a family: P = 4/5. Children will clear up with Hassan's help: P = 4/5. Do a breathing relaxation exercise in the lounge: A = 4/5; P = 3/5. Bedtime routine. Watch TV with Hassan for thirty minutes: P = 4/5.
night	Bed 9.30 p.m.

What happened for Razia with her Activity Plan and the experiment to change the daily routines:

Razia discovered that she was less tired with less pain and yet felt she was getting more done! She discovered she was less stressed in the mornings. Hassan's parents were understanding of her changes and the situation. She was also enjoying the time she spent with her family more. She decided to continue doing the activities that were important to her and still practising pacing with relaxation breaks.

Overall, she had a sense of achievement and more pleasure, while at the same time reducing how much she 'overdid it'. She felt less depressed by 30 per cent in the first week and more confident to manage.

EXPERIMENTING WITH THE ACTIVITY PLAN TOOL BELOW

This skill is to track your current activities through the day and night and then review them. This helps understand how the day and night are filled and if your activities and other things are in a balanced way to manage low moods and improve enjoyment. The next action is to then incorporate activities that help manage moods, so they are more enjoyable or pleasurable (P) or give a sense of achievement (A). It is also to reduce or change activities that are unhelpful or stressful.

For example: Razia stopped some of her daily visits to Hassan's parents and used the time for a relaxation break.

First action: Keep a record of what is happening each hour or two each day for at least **three days** in the activity planning sheet below. Is there anything you notice about what you do or the way you do it or think about it? Like 'unhelpful pacing patterns', 'guilt feelings', 'must do now thinking'.

Next action is to start planning your activities into the table below. Think about:

- what is most important to you;
- how to pace your activities and incorporate breaks;
- getting necessary things done;
- including enjoyable/fun activities;
- incorporating rewards into your plan.

ACTIVITY PLAN TO HELP MANAGE MOODS

→: page 373

Activity Plan	How to use an Activity Plan Track your activities through the day and night. Write them down and rate how much: • satisfaction or sense of achievement, with the scale range A = 0, no achievement, and 5 = maximum achievement; • enjoyment or pleasure, with the scale range P = 0, no pleasure at all, and 5 = extremely pleasurable; e.g. walked in the park: 2/5. TIP: When planning new activities, use a new sheet and focus on planning into each day: • a balance between getting necessary things done; • doing enjoyable or pleasurable activities that make you feel connected with others; • doing things that are an achievement or give you satisfaction; • pace yourself and the changes →: page 379.

Time of the day or night	Mon	Tue	Wed	Thu	Fri	Sat	Sun
a.m.							
p.m.							
evening							
night							

2. Learn to challenge automatic unhelpful thinking with the Four-Steps approach

In any situation, people try to make sense of what is happening by asking, 'Why me?' or 'What if?' With chronic pain, thoughts or beliefs about yourself, your health, and your ability to cope, may all be challenged.

When people are depressed, they sometimes end up thinking that they are useless or not needed. They may make assumptions, or have misbeliefs about what other people think, that are:

- usually negative;
- based on how they feel rather than on any evidence or facts.

Now check back to negative unhelpful thinking styles in Step 2 of the Four-Step Challenge to managing unhelpful thinking in moods → *: page 245.*

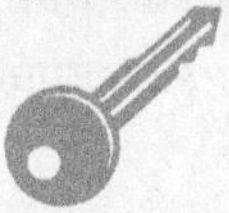

Thoughts about being helpless, hopeless, or not in control all impact on mood. In a low mood, our minds tend to remember difficult and negative experiences. The 'negative mental filter' switches in and so focus of thinking is much less on pleasant or positive thoughts. This unhelpful negative thinking shift makes the depressed feelings worse, and along with pain comes a vicious cycle that leads to us doing fewer kind actions that help to lessen low moods.

Once low mood sets in, these negative thoughts seem quite reasonable to us, and can get quite repetitive too.

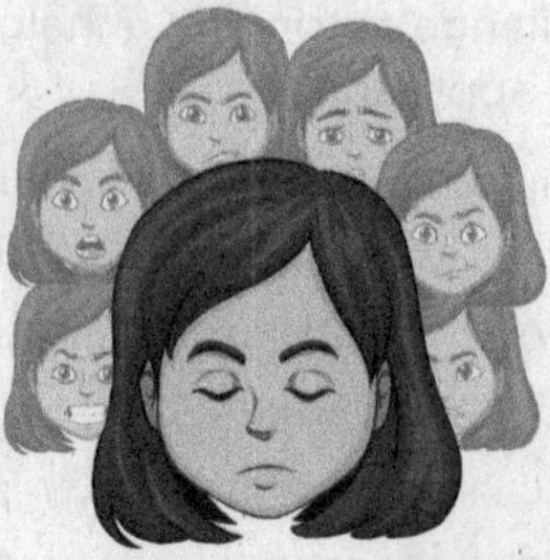

Review the thought challenge skills in the Managing anxiety, worry and fears chapter as this same set of skills are used to manage depressive unhelpful thinking →: page 248.

The Four Steps to Balanced Thinking to manage depressed moods:

Step 1: Start to notice thoughts and feelings (mood change) and use the Automatic Thought Tracker.

Step 2: Notice thoughts and unhelpful thinking styles (check thinking styles list →: page 245).

____

____

____

Step 3: Challenge your unhelpful thoughts and patterns; discover that they may not be 100 per cent true.

Decide how much you believe these thoughts are true in step 1. Give them a rating from 0–100 per cent (0 = not true; 100 per cent totally true).

Write down any evidence that **supports** these negative thoughts.

____

____

Write down any evidence that does **not support** 100 per cent these thoughts.

____

____

Think again about how much you believe the thoughts now. Has the rating changed?

____

____

Step 4: Develop and practise more balanced thoughts.

What would your best friend or someone who cares about you say if they knew of these negative thoughts or thinking styles?

____

____

What would you say to them if they had these or similar thoughts?

Are there any strengths or positives in you or the situation that you are ignoring?

Is there any kind or caring advice or support you would offer someone thinking in a similar way?

Rate your overall confidence level in balanced thinking (0 = no confidence and 100 per cent = totally confident).

0 1 2 3 4 5 6 7 8 9 10

Not at all confident — Extremely confident

3. Role of medicines for helping with depression

Anti-depressant medication is useful in managing depression. These medicines can help lessen your low mood with daily use. They usually take two to four weeks to have any positive effect and some may have a few side-effects at first. If you feel that medicines might be helpful, or if you have concerns about taking them, talk to your prescribing doctor.

If you do take anti-depressants, it is important to be consistent, and take them every day for at least six months to help improve depressed moods in the longer term. If you don't take the tablets regularly for several months, it will be difficult to know if they will really help you, or to see the real effect they have had on your depression.

It is always important to consult your doctor if you want to stop or reduce your medicines. Your doctor, pharmacist or other healthcare professionals will support you and answer questions about your medications.

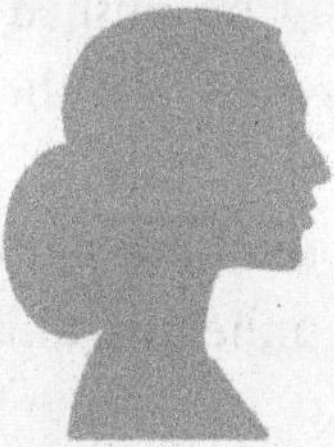

Razia discussed medication with her family doctor at her last appointment. Her doctor shared some options

to help, such as trying anti-depressant medicine and/or talking therapy. Razia talked it over with Hassan when she got home. She was not keen to try more medicines and Hassan just wanted her to feel better as soon as possible. They agreed that she would try some other ways of managing her moods first. If she didn't feel quite a bit better in the next six to eight weeks, she would try the anti-depressants and think more about talking therapy. Razia could see it might help and yet she wanted to try and manage herself now she understood much more about moods.

The value of a course of anti-depressant medicines is that they lift your mood and may help with sleep, so you can then help yourself to take action and use other options such as the following:

- Using an Activity Plan to improve day-to-day life. This planning can make sure you begin or continue activities that are creative, rewarding, pleasurable or calming/soothing to build more feelings of enjoyment. They can too easily be pushed out by daily life, by more pain and busyness, yet they contribute to better moods.
- Improve balanced thinking with the Four-Steps challenge to managing unhelpful thinking.

4. What to do if you feel hopeless or despairing about things and life

If your mood gets really low and you get to the point where you feel it isn't worth carrying on, or you have thoughts of hurting yourself or ending your life, it is really important to get help as soon as possible so you can keep yourself safe and feel better soon. There are good, trustworthy sources of help, 24 hours a day. Find out more →: page 355–6.

Feelings like this can happen when you have low mood or depression, and particularly when your situation is very difficult. These feelings and thoughts might go through your mind briefly from time to time, and get better if you follow your plan, or do something else.

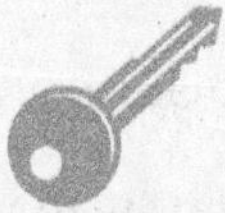

If you find that you keep on thinking that others would be better off without you, or start making plans to hurt yourself, please tell someone. If other people say that they are concerned about how low your mood is, or aren't sure that you are looking after yourself, this is another reason to get some extra support.

If you are able to speak to a trusted friend or family member, see if this helps. If you don't feel able to tell them everything about the thoughts you are having, it can still be helpful to talk to someone.

Make an appointment to see your family doctor or nurse. If you feel you can't keep yourself safe, you should get in touch with emergency services to ask for help.

If you have had these thoughts and feelings before, it's worth keeping a note of important things to remember, including contact details of friends or family members who are helpful; your doctor or the Samaritans; people who will listen without judging you.

You may find that it's difficult to take care of yourself or other people who depend on you. It can be hard to admit that you're struggling.

It is time to ask for help if you are at the point where you are neglecting yourself, drinking too much, or really can't look after others who need taking care of. Talking to someone you trust can be a good place to start. Check Resources ➔: page 355.

Resources and tools to support changes

Most of this book is about how to manage pain with greater confidence, and improve your quality of life as much as you can. It is also helpful to make some space for the feelings you have about the losses you've experienced. This is more about getting used to the changes that those losses bring, and accepting the feelings you have. It is not about ruminating or dwelling on things that we can't change.

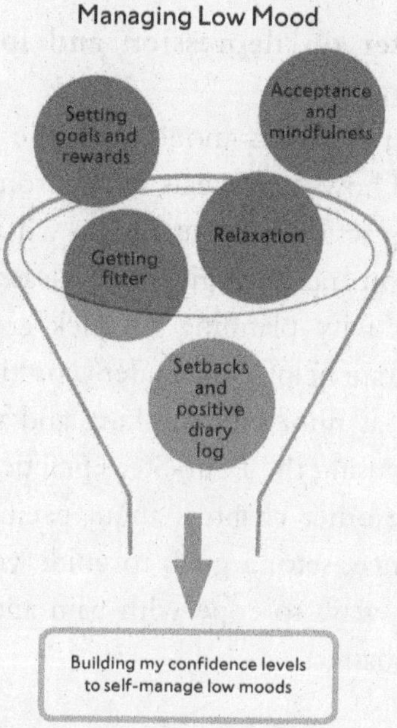

The chapter on Acceptance and moving on offers helpful ideas on dealing with painful emotions about situations we did not choose or plan to happen → : page 31.

Other chapters that may help with low mood are those dealing with values and acceptance, rewards, pacing, relaxation, mindfulness and dealing with setbacks. Check the contents page to find what section you need.

This chapter on depression and low moods explored ways:

- to understand this mood with the Five-Areas tool and how it connects with chronic pain;
- of taking action to focus and do what is important to you and what gives you pleasure in life;
- using activity planning to track activities and incorporate helpful or kinder activities;
- to look at unhelpful thinking and what to do about it using the Four-Steps practice;
- of using other chapters about pacing, rewards, acceptance, setting goals to guide you to more positive ways to cope with pain and unhelpful mood changes.

Important: Ideas in this book are about self-help. If you, or someone who cares about you, is concerned for your safety, including whether you are really able to look after yourself or others who depend on you, then do seek professional trusted help through our Resources pages ➔: page 355–6.

15

Managing setbacks and planning for the future

What this chapter covers

Hopefully, by exploring the other chapters of the book, you have had the chance to think about and experiment with helpful changes to live well and manage pain more confidently. So this chapter is about reviewing this journey to where you are now and ways to maintain what works well and continue your progress and success.

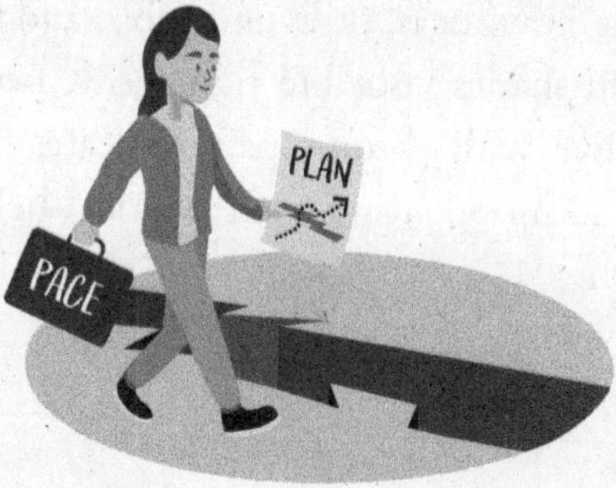

The chapter looks at where you would like to be in the future, and deals with the setbacks and challenges that happen along the way. There are some ideas on how to see them through with less suffering and distress, so keeping yourself on track to live well. It offers some ideas to map your future journey.

There are new skills to try, like problem solving everyday challenges and ways to shape your thinking style and approaches with a Positive Diary Log based on your progress and successes →: page 324.

Useful things to know about moving forward and keeping going

The chapters of the book have been written to give you more knowledge and confidence in managing the different five areas affected by your pain. It can be really empowering to explore the possibilities for helpful change, for example on your sleep, activity levels, work, pacing and moods. You may have noticed and continue to feel the benefits of working with some new ideas, skills and tools, and reducing the ways that pain shapes your life right now. Feedback from people who live with chronic pain indicates that, in time, over weeks and months, and with practice, helpful changes always happen.

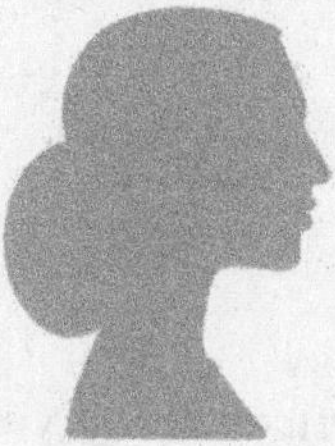

Razia learnt more about chronic pain and activity levels, and when she practised her pacing and relaxation skills, she found that she could achieve more around the house. Over six weeks she was able to spend more time outside, enjoying more fun times with Hassan and their sons in the local park.

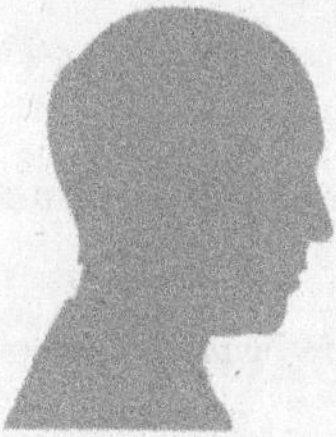

Jim discovered within four weeks that in actually trying to do a little less at a slower pace with more breaks, he achieved more overall, with less pain and less worry at the end. He even started to sleep better and was able to plan a treat with Anne to go to the garden centre for lunch.

What have you noticed about yourself since reading the other chapters and starting to make some links between what you are thinking, feeling, doing/not doing?

____

____

____

Have you been able to experiment with changes in any areas in the self-care cycle?

Changing the Impact of Pain

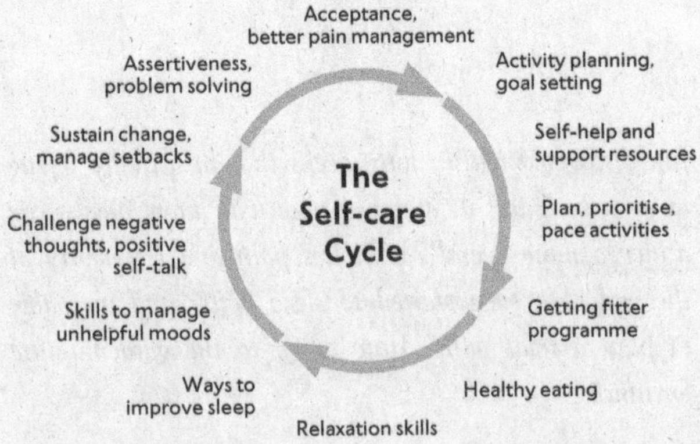

Circle those areas you have tried so far on the cycle and then write down what changes you find helpful and want to continue.

My valued changes to become confident to live well with pain are:

____

____

____

____

Planning the future

You may now believe it is time to focus on your goals more in the longer term and the range of possibilities open to you in the future. Hopefully you feel that you, and not the pain, are now in control of your life. Some people start to think about the next steps in their lives. For example, Jim loves walking, so he would like to become a community health walk leader in the future. He is now thinking about where to get some training.

Long-term goals may be about work that may be paid or unpaid. Some people decide on a career change, or plan a return to work or even reducing hours to ensure they continue in their current role. Some people, like Mo, may want to set some long-term physical activity goals, such as doing a park-run every Saturday or make plans to travel and discover different cultures and places. By setting SMART goals for short- and long-term and building in steps to achieve them, most things are possible given time, even when setbacks happen ➔: page 115.

You may find it helpful to record your progress, for example in a diary or blog, taking photos, or even making a short video so that you can look back and see how far you have come. Some people use a Positive Diary Log to record how they are managing with different aspects in their life **despite** pain.

How to create a Positive Diary Log to record your progress

You will need a diary or a small notepad or perhaps a mobile phone photo record. Some people use social media and set up a blog to record and share experiences. Here are some examples of how Mo and Razia did this.

It is important that the evidence means something to you. It can be evidence of more balanced thinking, making more helpful actions like pacing better, change in moods, so feeling more times of enjoyment.

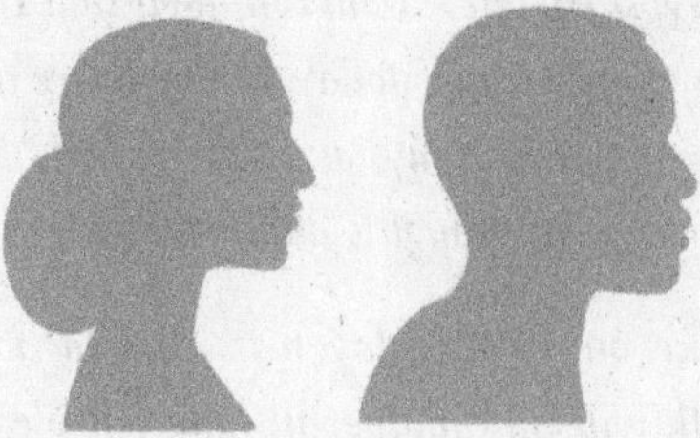

First step: *Razia and Mo each chose a sentence that most reflected the evidence of what they want to say each day about their positive changes. For example:*

Mo wrote that his evidence would be: 'that I can manage my pain and my life better because today . . .' and then he put in his proof for that day:

Monday: I got up at 8 a.m. now three days in a row.

Razia wrote that her evidence would be: 'I am confident that I am able to live with my pain because today . . .' and then she put in her evidence for that day:

Wednesday: I feel happy as I went for a walk in the park for fifteen minutes before the children came home.

Razia and Mo wrote the same evidence statement every day and then added a piece of evidence to this statement to show to themselves that it was true.

On Monday, Razia wrote: 'I am confident that I am able to live with my pain because today I went to meet the children from school: Proof of helpful action.'

On Tuesday, she wrote: 'I am confident that I am able to live with my pain because today I thought we could go for a family picnic on Sunday, and felt excited: More proof of helpful change in thoughts and feelings.'

Her evidence on Wednesday was: 'I had a short ten-minute walk with my mother-in-law; felt pleased: Proof of taking action and better feelings.'

Each statement builds into a record over time, and Razia looked back at all her evidence over two weeks. She was pleased about everything that she was achieving as a result of her planning and making priorities, problem solving and practice. Her confidence in her ability to manage her pain and her setbacks grew over time. She shared it with Hassan, and he saw it too and hugged her.

It is a skill worth trying and can be fun and creative. It helps the mind realise that the evidence shows the mind cannot **ignore a success or positive progress**, **dismiss it** as 'just done anyhow' or **discount** it as 'something little achieved'. Razia counted her ten-minute walk as progress because she knew she had only managed five minutes' walk the previous month. It made her think and feel more confident to focus on the present and all she was steadily achieving.

Mo found the same when he created a blog and showed pictures of his positive changes. Like climbing the stairs three times per day and he got positive comments from his friends and family. He put their positive comments as evidence in the blog too.

Problem solving for daily life challenges or issues

Problem-solving skills may help with extra life challenges or problems, some of which may or may not be due to having chronic pain. For example, how to tackle a household task such as who is going to paint the hall, the washing machine has packed in, or a child is ill and off school.

Problem-solving skills help so that you are not side-tracked repeatedly and are able to continue making progress with your goals and stay confident.

Using a step-by-step problem-solving approach may help you to work out if something is changeable or not. The acceptance that a problem is not always changeable may be helpful in dealing with the emotions and thoughts when you realise this and adjust.

The Five Steps to Problem Solving

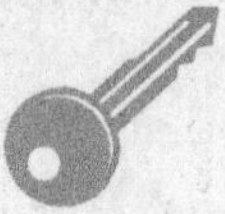

Step 1: Recognise and define the problem

Step 2: Make a list of all possible solutions

Step 3: List all the possible advantages and disadvantages of each idea

Step 4: Choose the best solution

Step 5: Review your progress

Step 1: Recognise and define the problem

Acknowledge there is a problem and be clear exactly what the problem is. This helps to decide if you can, or want to, do something about it. It will buy you some time to consider your options. Sometimes it helps to talk to a few different people about it.

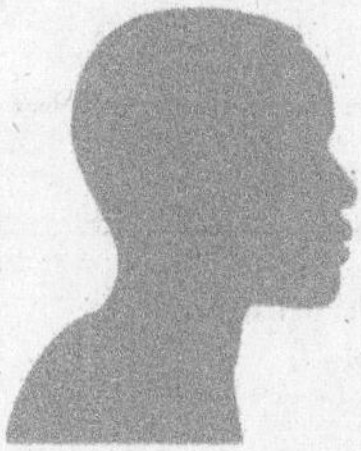

Step 1: What is my problem? Mo ask's himself.

> *'Mo's problem . . . getting fed-up and frustrated with being stuck in the house most days.'*

Step 2: What are my options for solutions?

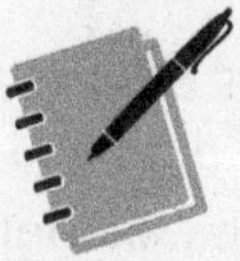

These are ideas about how to solve the problem – they might be 'funny', 'silly' or even 'bad' suggestions; try not to limit yourself at this stage. Mo even thought about getting a skateboard to 'whizz around on in the lounge'!

Step 3: What are all the possible advantages and disadvantages of each option?

This may help you to see what is really 'do-able' and what is not. Discussing these with family and friends can be fun and often a clear solution emerges →: page 212.

MO'S SOLUTIONS

Idea	*Advantages*	*Disadvantages*
Skateboard	*Could get around quickly*	*I don't even own a skateboard; it'd upset the dog*
Juggling balls	*Easy and cheap to buy, fun, helps with concentration*	*Do not know where to get them*

Step 4: Make a decision about the best solution and take action

From your list choose the solution that you are most likely/able to carry out. It may not be the perfect answer, but it is worth a try. Stick with the solution you decide on and give it a go, like an experiment. Review it later and if it didn't work, choose the next thing to try from your list.

Step 5: Review your progress

How did it go, what went well, what didn't go so well, what will I try next?

Hopefully things went to plan and you managed to work around a problem with the solution you chose. If things didn't work out as planned, you may need to think over options for change or try a different suggestion. *And* you have discovered how not to solve the problem that way! This turns out often to be truly valuable to learn from it. Thomas Edison, who experimented to create an electric light bulb, discovered how to make one successfully and 999 ways how not to make one!!

Mo's solution: He decided to learn how to juggle and do more activity around the house to build up his strength and balance so that he would be more confident when going out on his own.

Rewards help you to repeat success

Plan small and give yourself rewards often and in different ways. This could be each day, each week, or when you have achieved one of your short-term goals. Working to a specific reward can be very motivational for some people and planning the reward can be fun. Get creative when thinking about your rewards and discuss them with others. A reward could be afternoon tea with a friend, a drive in the country, a game of crazy golf, or an extra five-minute snooze. It doesn't have to cost money; you could take a walk in the park, for example, to see the bluebells, or could just sit in the sun: simply feel and listen to the experience →: page 110.

Rewarding yourself gives you the opportunity to think about how far you have come, as well as to dream, plan and share your next goal.

How will setback planning help with managing chronic pain?

The reality of life is that it rarely runs smoothly without

any hitches or challenges; setbacks do and will happen from time to time.

A setback is a disruption or hitch interfering with what you have planned or with a goal that you have set and are working on. Sometimes a setback can be predicted; sometimes, like a flat tyre, it appears 'out of the blue'.

If we accept that setbacks happen along the way, perhaps getting in the way of you achieving your SMART goals →: page 115, or of the daily walk, or of the visit to the cinema you promised yourself, then a plan for dealing with them is really helpful. Being prepared for a setback may result in:

- reducing the fear or frustration it can bring;
- the setback lasting for a shorter time;
- the setback being less severe;
- others close to you knowing how to support better.

Planning how to respond to a setback can be helpful, both in the short term and the longer term.

The skill is to create a setback plan to have ready to stay in control and minimise the impact of a setback. It helps to focus on key areas that are likely to be affected by a setback, small or big. The setback plan could use these areas to focus on. Whatever the actions they need to be SMART Specific, Measurable, Achievable, Realistic and Timed. The actions maybe start with an activity at a slow level then build it up, e.g. taking a walk for fifteen minutes for days one to three, then increase to thirty minutes for days four to seven and so on.

Some examples are given from Mo's setback plans and ways to stay active as the setback settled.

Mo's setback plan:

- to manage the pain, e.g. *do longer relaxation breaks in the morning and evening at 9 p.m.*
- if worried and tense about the setback, e.g. *'tell myself they always settle in a week and pace it'*;
- to stay physically active, e.g. *cut back on stretches to about half and same with walks up the street, not to the shops*;
- to deal with 'catastrophic' negative thinking, e.g. *Mo thought what would Paul my friend say to me . . . 'they happen and they settle quicker than you think'*;
- to sleep well even during the setback, e.g. *listen to my audiobook when I wake in the night, it helps me back to sleep*;
- to ask for help and support, e.g. *show my dad the plan and talk about what he and Mum can do . . . no fussing, remind me about relaxation time*;
- to work out my priorities of what needs to be done, e.g. *need to work on this.*

A setback plan helps you to stay confident so that you can manage the setback. Share the plan with others who support you as they know what they can do to be really useful. The plan can keep yourself and others grounded in times of stress. It can then reduce the worry or stress for everybody and help turn down the amount of pain.

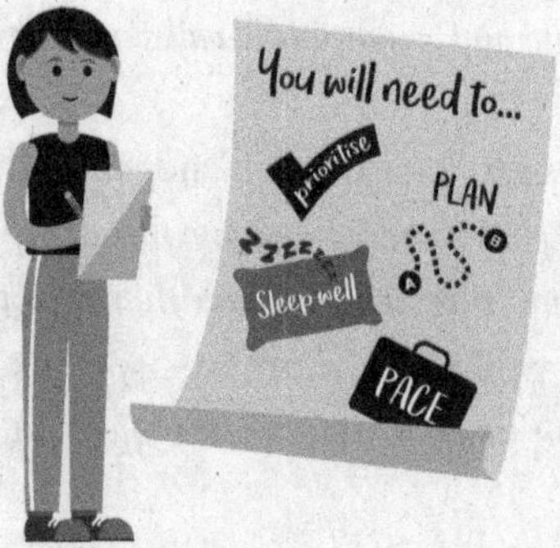

Building your setback plan so as to be confident to manage setbacks

People with pain who have experienced setbacks tell us that they simply have to stay on the first or basic activity for a week or so until they are ready to move on. Think of the walking example above. Let's take a look at what Mo did when he got flu in his setback plan → : page 335.

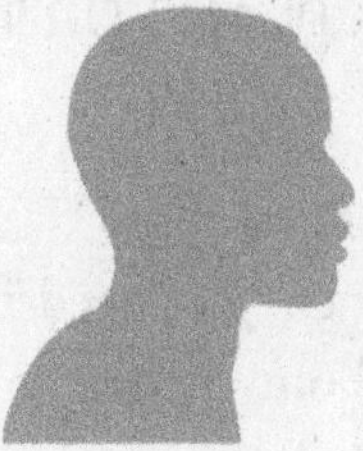

MO'S SETBACK PLAN FOR KEEPING ACTIVE

Mo was doing his twenty-minute walk four times a week, at a moderate pace, without stopping. Then he got flu and could not walk outdoors for a week. When he improved, he decided that, as he was feeling weak and tired, he would reduce the walk time to ten minutes for the first week. Then he built up to fifteen minutes over the next two weeks. He found that by doing this he managed to continue with four walks each week. He then built things up slowly, and at four weeks he had increased his walk time to twenty-five minutes, with a stop. He went to see a new film at the cinema with his friend Paul as a treat and was starting to think, 'Okay, I've got this, what next? Perhaps sign up at the local gym.'

YOUR SETBACK PLAN FOR THE NEXT FEW DAYS OR WEEK OR TWO

It may help to write yourself a setback plan that is easy to look at when you need it. Perhaps keep it on your mobile phone or on the refrigerator or by your bed.

These are some ideas from others living with chronic pain:

- Keep as gently active as you are able around the house.
- Cut down the time spent standing, walking and sitting by half for the first few days.
- Do stretches, cut down the number and aim to do three times a day.
- Listen to music or other soothing things.
- Tackle a list of enjoyable activities, e.g. make the model train, do that easy jigsaw, watch that 'fun movie' with the grandkids, plan a holiday.
- Practise relaxed breathing more often through the day.
- Look back on your Positive Diary Log: 'The last three weeks have been good and I will get back on track very soon.' This helps you develop your own positive coping self-talk.
- Be kind to yourself: 'We all have bad days and setbacks and I have a plan.'
- Realise that a setback passes and better times are ahead.

- Look for the positives: 'At least I got to finish my book' or 'Got the vegetable seeds planted up'.

When writing your plan of what to do when you have a setback, think and plan in the following areas.

1. **Physical activities:** Think about what to reduce, how much, for how long, and when to increase it again, perhaps in a similar way to Mo's plan above.
2. **Enjoyable activities:** List things that would be enjoyable and rewarding to do. Razia loved to watch 'a family fun movie' after a warm bath with aromatherapy oils.
3. **Tasks, around the house, in the garden, at work, with family, involving social activities:** Think about priorities and pacing, including more breaks, asking for help. Razia asked Hassan to help put out the bin and do some of the heavy shopping.
4. **Relaxation:** Explore relaxation or mindfulness practices that work easily and well for you in a setback. Jim found listening to 'waves of the seashore and belly breathing helpful and did it more often after tasks in the house'.

In my setback plan I will try (use the above headings):

1. ______________________________

____

____

2. ______________________________

____

____

3. ______________________________

____

____

Now you have a setback plan how **confident** are you that you **can manage the next** setback?

0 1 2 3 4 5 6 7 8 9 10

Not at all confident Extremely confident

If your confidence is low (less than 5), then review your plan →: page 336, and use the question 'What would my best friend suggest to improve my setback plan?'

Tips to support change

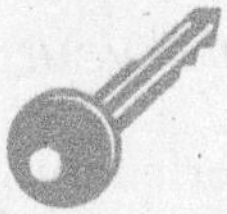

Sometimes people with chronic pain struggle with looking to the future. They are not sure how to keep moving forward and making progress. Here are a few things that people with chronic pain have suggested about keeping going and moving forward:

- Make short- and long-term goals.
- Review your progress often.
- Keep a record of your progress, like the Positive Diary Log, journal or a blog. Check it regularly to remind yourself how far you've come.
- Each time you have a setback, review your setback plan and ask yourself: is this still the right plan for me? If not, adjust it. This is all good progress.
- Address your problems using the five stages of problem solving.
- Add to your fitness plan and make sure the activities are enjoyable for you.
- Reward yourself often and well.

Self-check on progress and making plans

The ongoing journey and your future

Over the last twenty years, more research has supported the value of pain self-management. Using a person-centred Five-Areas tool really works, and developments in talking therapies mean that there are more choices and improved ways of getting help and support. As with a bus journey, the timetable and the route can change, and it is worth exploring these approaches further to guide and support your ongoing journey.

In the long run, people who have learnt pain self-management, either in groups or individually, have fewer mood problems, including being less depressed and enjoying

Life Plan Versus Reality

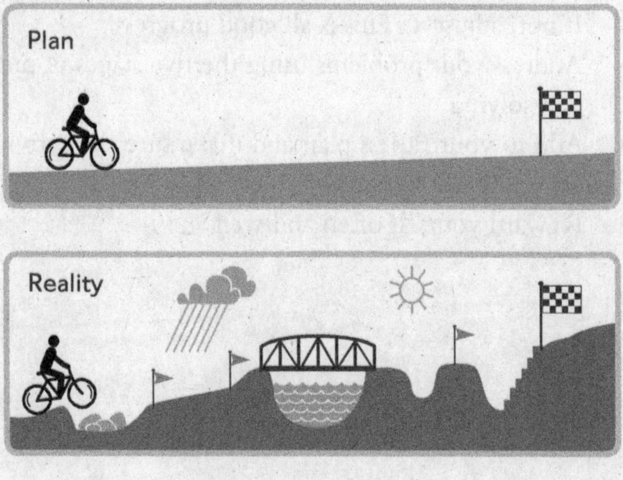

better sleep. They are more active, more creative, enjoy work, and overall have a better quality of life despite living with chronic pain.

They also know that the journey is not a straight line; the reality is a journey of diversions, slip-ups and exciting golden life moments.

Some suggestions to guide the ongoing life journey

Acceptance and mindfulness enable you to focus the mind in more helpful, grounded ways ➔: page 31. Instead of paying attention mostly to pain, stress, difficult moods, situations or people, it is possible to learn and practise a different, kinder approach. Mindfulness helps the mind to be like an observer, and just notice these things, without being 'sucked in' or stuck on them.

Hurt and pain need soothing, kindness, and care for ourselves and others. You can benefit from knowing more of this compassionate approach, both now and in the future journeys of life.

Research shows that approaches to self-care that focus on compassionate meditation practice can help the heart and mind of the person become more peaceful and happy ➔: Resources page 349. These 'loving-kindness' or compassion actions towards oneself and others help the brain to turn down the volume on pains of all types. Actively being soothing and compassionate to oneself and others calms the emotional areas of the brain that deal with anxiety, threat and anger. This means that less adrenaline is released into the system, and so fewer threat reactions happen. At the same time, this kind of self-compassion practice increases the brain's own soothing and calming centres. More of the natural opioid chemicals are released, which in turn helps wind down the person's pain, hurt and distress within themselves and their body.

An example of a 'loving-kindness' practice is shared here. This kind of practice for pain or any other struggle means that we move from *anxious attention* by the mind and heart to the threats of pain or struggle, to *loving attention* within the mind and the heart. The idea is to intend to be kind, loving and compassionate to the suffering and distress. This, with practice, leads to a kinder way to be open to pain, rather than pushing or fighting against its existence. This leads towards a greater sense of peace and well-being within.

LOVING-KINDNESS: A GUIDED MEDITATION SCRIPT

This meditation is about focusing on the 'feeling' of loving-kindness. We use words to guide the learning of loving-kindness meditation, but the words are not the main point. Over time, the words can fade and you'll simply be left with the feeling. That itself is the overall aim.

1. SIT QUIETLY AND COMFORTABLY

- Sit in a comfortable way but without being in a sleepy position.
- For example, sit with your back straight, head up, feet on the floor and your arms gently in your lap.
- Simply sit and notice yourself in sitting, letting go of any tension in the body.
- Breathe naturally.
- In your mind's eye, watch your breath going in and your breath going out. Keep focusing on your breathing for a while.

2. PLACE YOUR ATTENTION ON THE AREA AROUND YOUR HEART

Gently place your attention on the area in the middle of your chest, around your heart. Perhaps place your right hand over your heart area.

Repeat to yourself gently and softly, feeling the resonance of the words:

'Just as all beings wish to be happy and free from suffering, may I be happy and free from suffering.'

As you say this, if you like, bring to mind something that you feel caring and loving towards.

It may be an image of a soft, lovable dog, or the

serene look on someone's face, or a baby, or the feeling of the soft fur as you stroke a kitten . . .

This image is simply to help you kick-start the feelings.

If a feeling of loving-kindness arises without these images, there is no need for them.

3. EXPERIENCE FEELING LOVE THROUGH YOUR WHOLE BODY

Let yourself feel the warmth of that loving attention. Feel the sense of caring, healing and soothing. Let it wash over you and through you while you gently repeat silently to yourself:

- 'May I be safe.
- May I be happy.
- May I be healthy.
- May I live in ease.'

Sometimes people find this stage difficult to do at first. So take your time, repeat one word or phrase a few times to fully absorb the meaning. Should you feel lost, just return to these phrases.

It may be helpful to spend some days or weeks simply cultivating loving-kindness for yourself. Fifteen to twenty minutes most days can help this skill develop well. There is no need to rush, as it is developing the quality of feeling that matters.

Explore the Resources →: page 352, where you will find ideas for written and audio access to this compassion-focused approach.

Loving-kindness practice does not directly change how we feel. We now understand the more focus we make on doing more kindness and caring actions helps emotions, including painful ones, to change, gradually becoming less hurtful and more positive. With each kind word to yourself, you are planting a seed that will grow and blossom into good feelings; this means being less anxious and less upset or pained when things go wrong. Explore Resources →: page 349.

Being part of activities and experiences

It may be an important step to take to become part of activities that have a common focus and offer support, friendship and the chance to contribute to local communities or neighbourhoods as well. Jim realised that he would like to become a community walk leader and be part of the local health walks group. So, become creative and adventurous and try a range of things that are of interest or are enjoyable. Examples are knitting and craft groups, felting and picture making, t'ai chi, yoga, model making, learning a new skill and so on. Birdwatching is increasingly being thought of as 'bird therapy' for its benefits as a mindful, kindly activity. Remember to explore the ten keys to happier living and make it happen to yourself.

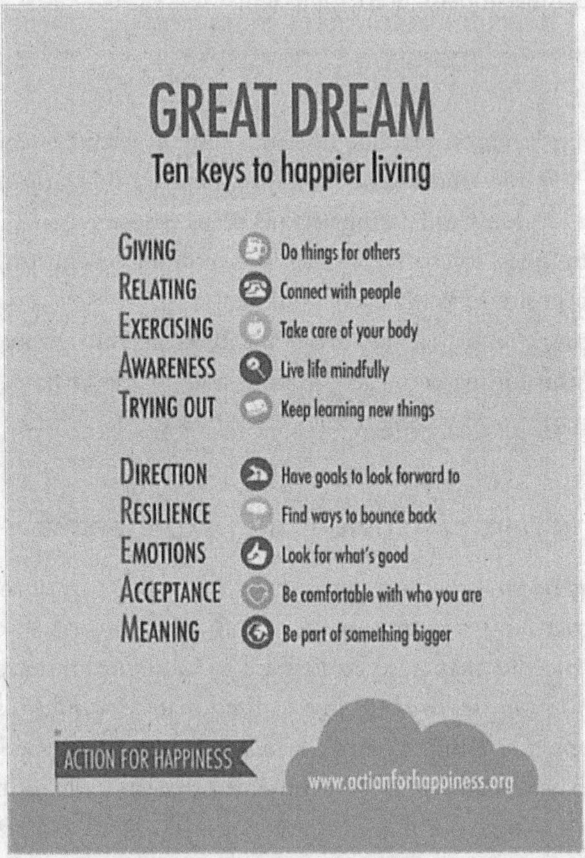

Chapter summary

- It's helpful to keep looking and moving forward, knowing changes are possible over time with SMART goals. Short- and long-term goal setting helps you to live well despite pain.
- Keeping a simple record of your evidence of positive progress as a Positive Diary Log is a neat way of developing self-confidence in your skills and ability to manage well. It guides your thinking to be aware of the evidence of thinking, feeling, and the actions that you take, or the experiences every day that are true achievements and successes.
- Setbacks always happen. A plan helps you to get back on track quicker and builds confidence in managing the next one.
- Problem-solving skills mean that you gain more positive control over your life situation. The Five Steps are a useful guide to work with and review.
- Rewarding yourself can be fun and helps with motivation.
- Journeying into your future may mean exploring more about being compassionate through key meditation practices and skills including loving-kindness.

The best of journeys to you, and may you be safe, be happy and live life well.

Resources

This section contains information sources and organisations. These can offer support and information about a range of chronic pain conditions and ways to manage them.

Websites

Age UK

Online resources for ageing and being active.
www.ageuk.org.uk/services/in-your-area/exercise

Being Assertive: A Self-help Guide

Self-help on better communication by being more assertive.
www.moodjuice.scot.nhs.uk/assertiveness.asp

Body in Mind

www.bodyinmind.org

Breathworks

Offers a range of resources and practical support to build regular mindfulness practice and relaxation skills.
www.breathworks-mindfulness.co.uk

British Pain Society

Professional organisation with information for people with pain. Explore the 'people with pain' section and publications on medications and treatments.

www.britishpainsociety.org.uk

Chartered Society of Physiotherapy

Their Love Activity Hate Exercise campaign gives expert physiotherapy advice on getting more active. They also have information busting myths about back pain.

www.csp.org.uk/public-patient/keeping-active-and-healthy/love-activity-hate-exercise-campaign

www.csp.org.uk/public-patient/back-pain-myth-busters

GetSelfHelp

Self-help on better communication by being more assertive.

www.getselfhelp.co.uk/ccount/click.php?id=36

Go4Life

Information on how being active helps as we get older, from the National Institute on Aging.

www.go4life.nia.nih.gov/how-exercise-helps

Healthtalk

People with pain talk about their experiences, and also about goal setting, pacing, exercise and activity.

www.healthtalk.org/peoples-experiences/chronic-health-issues/chronic-pain/overview

www.healthtalk.org/peoples-experiences/long-term-conditions/chronic-pain/pain-management-pacing-and-goal-setting

www.healthtalk.org/peoples-experiences/long-term-conditions/chronic-pain/exercise-and-activity-chronic-pain

Live Well with Pain

Free-to-use resource supporting self-management of long-term pain, with online leaflets and resources linked into this *Overcoming Chronic Pain* book.
www.my.livewellwithpain.co.uk

MIND

The mental health charity. A valuable resource of web-based information and local support services, including for pain in some areas. There are online courses on coping with moods, relaxation and mindfulness.
www.mind.org.uk

My Cuppa Jo

It is a personal website by a person living with persistent pain and Jo uses scientific information and user-friendly language to bridge the gap between pain science and personal experience.
www.mycuppajo.com

National Sleep Foundation

The Natural Sleep Foundation has a wide range of

information about sleep, which includes how health issues can affect sleep. There are educational materials and exercises to help people sleep well.
www.sleepfoundation.org

NHS
NHS advice on managing long-term pain.
www.nhs.uk/live-well/healthy-body/ways-to-manage-chronic-pain

NHS – Avon Partnership Occupational Health
Information on communication, assertiveness and mental health.
www.apohs.nhs.uk/advice/mental-health/assertiveness

NHS – Change for Life
NHS resource for getting more active.
www.nhs.uk/change4life/activities

NHS – Get Fit for Free
NHS resources with ideas on getting free exercise and information on the benefits.
www.nhs.uk/live-well/exercise/free-fitness-ideas
www.nhs.uk/live-well/exercise/exercise-health-benefits

NHS – Northumberland, Tyne and Wear
An excellent collection of CBT resources for moods, anxiety, anger, depression, sleep and many other mind health areas.
www.ntw.nhs.uk/pic/selfhelp

Pain Association Scotland
www.painassociation.com

Pain Concern
Resources for people who have pain, including information and advice on sexual relationships.
www.painconcern.org.uk

Pain-Ed
Patient stories.
www.pain-ed.com/public/patient-stories-2

Pain Health
Information on pacing, goal setting and personal experiences.
www.painhealth.csse.uwa.edu.au/pain-module/pacing-and-goal-setting

The Pain Toolkit
Online leaflets and ebook developed by an expert patient in collaboration with pain clinicians. Twelve steps to self-managing your pain, and advice on pacing.
www.paintoolkit.org/resources/for-patients
www.paintoolkit.org/pain-tools/pacing

Self-compassion
Useful resource to discover ways to be kinder and more supportive to oneself with pain.
www. self-compassion.org

The Sleep Council

Provides helpful advice and tips on how to improve sleep quality.
www.sleepcouncil.org.uk

The Sleep School

Offers access to online courses and workshops to help you sleep better. Sessions are delivered by a sleep specialists team led by Dr Guy Meadows.
www.thesleepschool.org/insomnia

Sleepio

Linked with Colin Espie's *Overcoming* book (below), the website provides access to tools and techniques developed by experts that are proven to improve sleep.
www.sleepio.com/cbt-for-insomnia

Stitchlinks

Resources for people with pain and health problems to understand and get started in knitting and other activities.
www.stitchlinks.com

Veterans Pain Management Programme

www.bit.ly/2E3p03C

Self-help Groups and Organisations

Big White Wall

Online supportive community to help deal with depression and other mood difficulties.

www.bigwhitewall.com

Campaign Against Living Miserably (CALM)

Helpline and online resources campaigning to support men and prevent male suicide.

Call 0800 58 58 58 – 5 p.m. to midnight every day or visit the webchat page.

www.thecalmzone.net

IMAlive

Instant messaging chat crisis counselling with trained volunteers. Available to visitors from anywhere worldwide.

www.imalive.org

NHS – Suicidal Thoughts

NHS resources with help for suicidal thoughts.

www.nhs.uk/conditions/suicide

Papyrus

Suicide prevention and help for people under thirty-five.

Call 0800 068 41 41 – Monday to Friday 10 a.m. to 10 p.m., weekends 2 p.m. to 10 p.m., bank holidays 2 p.m. to 5 p.m.

Text: 07786 209697

Email: pat@papyrus-uk.org

Relate

Organisation focused on relationships, providing education, counselling and support.
www.relate.org.uk

Samaritans

Confidential listening service for everyone who is struggling or suicidal.
Call 116 123
www.samaritans.org

SANE Mental Health Helpline

Helpline for people experiencing mental health difficulties.
www.sane.org.uk

The Silver Line

Helpline for older adults.
Call 0800 4 70 80 90
www.thesilverline.org.uk

Self-help Books and Audio Resources

Living Beyond your Pain: Using Acceptance and Commitment Therapy to Ease Chronic Pain, J. Dahl (2006), New Harbinger.

A practical book on managing your pain using acceptance and commitment therapy approaches.

Living with Chronic Pain

This audio shares ways to manage pain and how to relax your body. It guides relaxation practice. Free MP3 audio download or CD to buy online.
www.paincd.org.uk

Mindfulness for Health: A Practical Guide to Relieving Pain, Reducing Stress and Restoring Wellbeing, V. Burch and D. Penman (2013), Piatkus.

A guide to increasing your well-being using meditation techniques.

The Mindfulness Journal, C. Sweet (2014), Boxtree.

A really useful resource to help you practically use mindfulness every day.

Overcoming Insomnia and Sleep Problems, C. Espie (2006), Robinson.

A self-help book based on the best evidence for improving your sleep.

The Pain Management Plan: A Practical Work Book on How People with Pain Found a Better Life with Pain
Evidence-based NHS workbook for pain management, with a CD. The relaxation programme CD guides relaxing the body and mind and so helps with better sleep.
www.pain-management-plan.co.uk

The Sleep Book, G. Meadows (2014), Orion.

Sleeping with Pain, S. Peacock (2016), Ann Jaloba.

Apps

CALM
App aimed at promoting better sleep and using meditation.
www.calm.com

Couch to 5K
A 'How to' guide to running from scratch.
www.c25k.com

My Fitness Pal
Advice, tracking and support for diet and fitness.
www.myfitnesspal.com

NHS – Recommended Health Apps
NHS online library of apps that are aimed at helping to improve health.
www.nhs.uk/apps-library

Walking Apps
A selection of free apps on walking.
www.verywellfit.com/best-walking-app-p2-3434995

Video Resources
Exercise advice videos.
www.csp.org.uk/public-patient/keeping-active-and-healthy/exercise-advice-videos

How Does your Brain Respond to Pain?, Karen Davies.
Helps with understanding how the brain responds to pain.
www.youtube.com/watch?v=I7wfDenj6CQ&sns=em

How Mindfulness Can Help Cope with Pain, Vidyamala Burch.
Shows how mindfulness can help cope with pain.
www.youtube.com/watch?v=iSGsTWcofhM

Pain and Me
Video on acceptance, with Tamar Pincus.
http://www.my.livewellwithpain.co.uk/resources/video-and-audio/pain-and-me

Understanding Pain in Five Minutes
Invaluable to make sense of persistent pain.
https://www.youtube.com/watch?v=5KrUL8tOaQs

Walking – 23 and ½ hours
www.youtube.com/watch?v=3F5Sly9JQao

Walking for Health
www.walkingforhealth.org.uk

Why Things Hurt, Lorimer Moseley
A TedX Talk from Adelaide in which an expert explains why we experience pain.
www.youtube.com/watch?v=gwd-wLdIHjs

Appendix

This appendix includes the following resource tools:

1. Five-Areas tool
2. Daily diary: my typical day (getting fitter pacing and goat setting)
3. SMART Goal Steps
4. Sleep diary
5. Automatic Thought Tracker and Four Step Thought Challenge
6. Activity plan to help manage moods
7. Problem-solving steps
8. Suggested sexual positions for chronic pain sufferers
9. Guide to safe medicine use
10. Setback plan
11. Pleasurable activity list

Copies of many of these tools can be found online at www.overcoming.co.uk and www.my.livewellwithpain.co.uk

1. Five-Areas tool

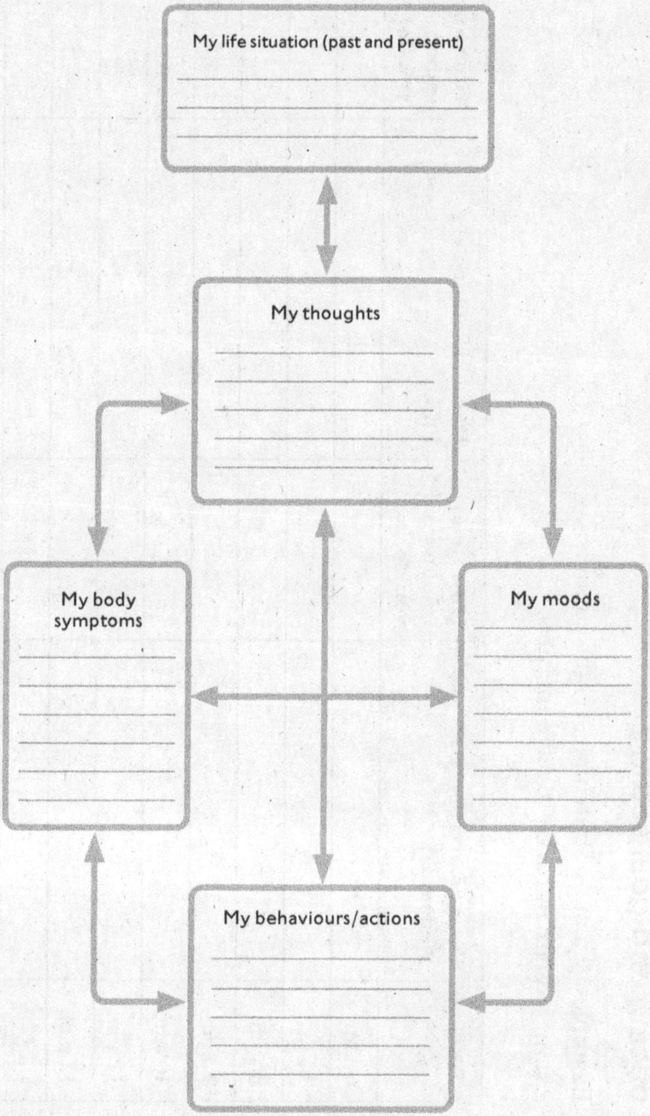

2. Daily diary: to track a typical day's activities to help with getting fitter, pacing and goal setting

Examples: 9 a.m. – Stretching – eight minutes.

2 p.m. – Walk in park – twelve minutes.

Time	Day and activity, e.g. Wednesday	How many minutes did you do?	Day and activity, e.g. Friday	How many minutes did you do?
6 a.m.				
7 a.m.				
8 a.m.				
9 a.m.				
10 a.m.				
11 a.m.				
12 p.m.				
1 p.m.				
2 p.m.				

3 p.m.				
4 p.m.				
5 p.m.				
6 p.m.				
7 p.m.				
8 p.m.				
9 p.m.				
10 p.m.				
11 p.m.				
12 a.m.				
1 a.m.				
2 a.m.				
3 a.m.				
4 a.m.				
5 a.m.				

3. SMART Goal Steps

My SMART goal at the end of ____________ weeks is to

____

My Goal Ladder

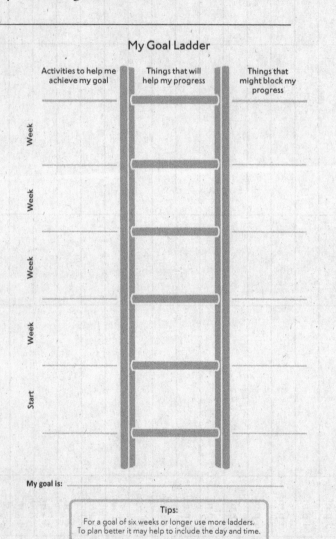

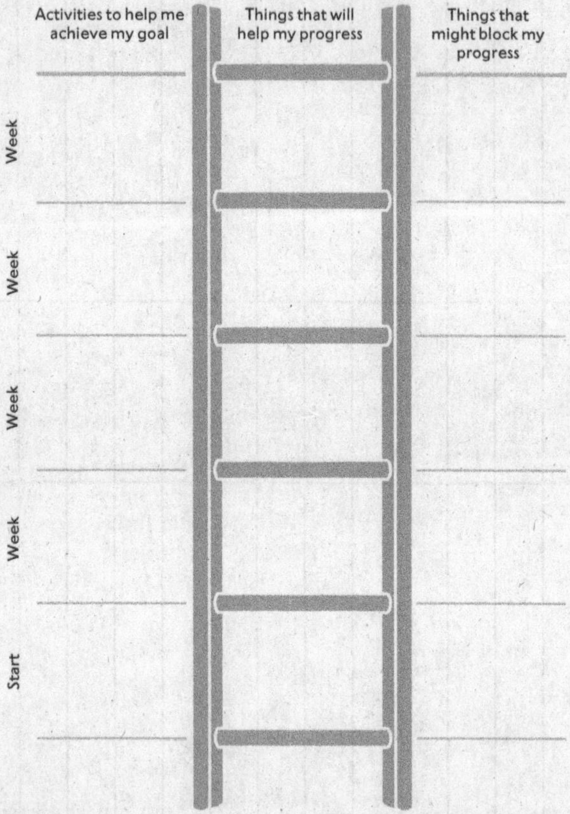

My goal is: ______________________________

Tips:

For a goal of six weeks or longer use more ladders.
To plan better it may help to include the day and time.

4. Sleep diary

Fill this in for at least a week and make a note of:

- where you were when you were asleep – **shade it in**;
- when you took medicines for pain or sleep;
- whether anything seemed to keep you awake.

Time	Mon	Tue	Wed	Thu	Fri	Sat	Sun
6 a.m.							
7 a.m.							
8 a.m.							
9 a.m.							
10 a.m.							
11 a.m.							
12 p.m.							
1 p.m.							
2 p.m.							
3 p.m.							
4 p.m.							
5 p.m.							

6 p.m.							
7 p.m.							
8 p.m.							
9 p.m.							
10 p.m.							
11 p.m.							
12 a.m.							
1 a.m.							
2 a.m.							
3 a.m.							
4 a.m.							
5 a.m.							

Once you have done the diary for several days or a week, what do you notice? It can be useful to make a note of any patterns, or things that seem to help. What would you like to try to change? Explore ideas in the Sleeping well chapter and try them out.

5. Automatic Thought Tracker and Four Steps to balanced thinking

Automatic Thought Tracker for use in Step 1.
Four Steps for challenging unhelpful thoughts.

Specific situation **What were you doing?** **Where?** **When?** **Who with?**	**Immediate thoughts and negative predictions** **Belief level in these thoughts** **0–100% (where 0 = none and 100% = totally)**	**Feelings, mood** **How bad was the feeling, on a scale of 0–100% (where 100% is the worst possible)?**	**Body symptoms felt**

The Four Steps for challenging unhelpful thoughts to achieve balanced thinking

Step 1: Start to notice thoughts and feelings; use the Automatic Thought Tracker as your mood changes.

Step 2: Notice unhelpful thinking styles (check thinking styles list →: page 246).

Step 3: Challenge your unhelpful thoughts and patterns; discover that they may not be 100 per cent true

- Decide how much you believe these thoughts in step 1 are true. Give them a rating from 0 to 100 per cent (0 = not true; 100 per cent totally true).

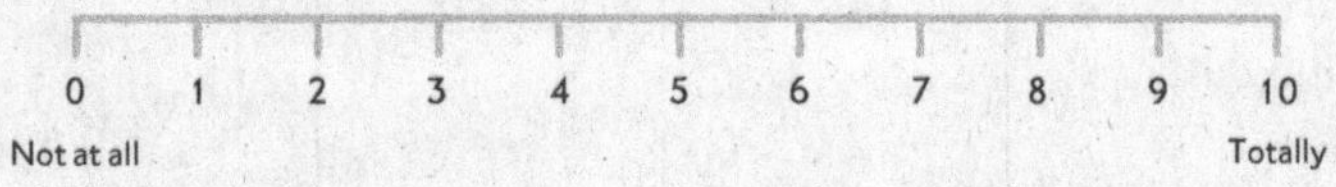

- Write down any evidence that **supports** these unhelpful negative thoughts.

- Write down any evidence that does **not support** these unhelpful thoughts 100 per cent.

- Think again about how much you believe the automatic thoughts. Has the rating changed?

Step 4: Develop and practise more balanced helpful thoughts

- What would your best friend or someone who cares for you say if they knew of these automatic negative thoughts?

- What would you say to them if they had these or similar unhelpful thoughts?

- Are there any strengths or positives in you or the situation that you are ignoring?

Write your balanced thoughts here.

Rate your overall **confidence** level in this balanced thinking (0 to 100 per cent)

0 1 2 3 4 5 6 7 8 9 10

Not at all confident — Extremely confident

6. Activity plan to help manage moods

➔ : page 306

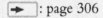

Activity Plan	How to use an Activity Plan Track your activities through the day and night. Write them down and rate how much: • satisfaction or sense of achievement, with the scale range A = 0, no achievement, and 5 = maximum achievement; • enjoyment or pleasure, with the scale range P = 0, no pleasure at all, and 5 = extremely pleasurable. TIP: When planning new activities, use a new sheet and focus on planning into each day: • a balance between getting necessary things done; • doing enjoyable or pleasurable activities that make you feel connected with others; • doing things that are an achievement or give you satisfaction; • pace yourself and the changes. ➔ : page 125.

Time of the day or night	Mon	Tue	Wed	Thu	Fri	Sat	Sun
a.m.							
p.m.							
evening							
night							

7. Problem-solving steps

Five Steps to Problem Solving

Step 1: Recognise and define the problem

Step 2: Make a list of all possible solutions

Step 3: List all the possible advantages and disadvantages of each idea

Step 4: Choose the best solution

Step 5: Review your progress

8. Suggested sexual positions for chronic pain sufferers

Old positions may not work for you if you have pain. Here are some suggestions to try.

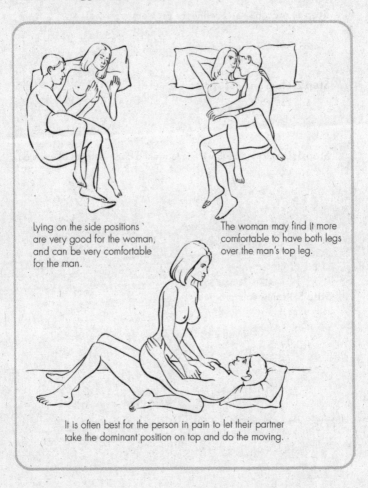

Lying on the side positions are very good for the woman, and can be very comfortable for the man.

The woman may find it more comfortable to have both legs over the man's top leg.

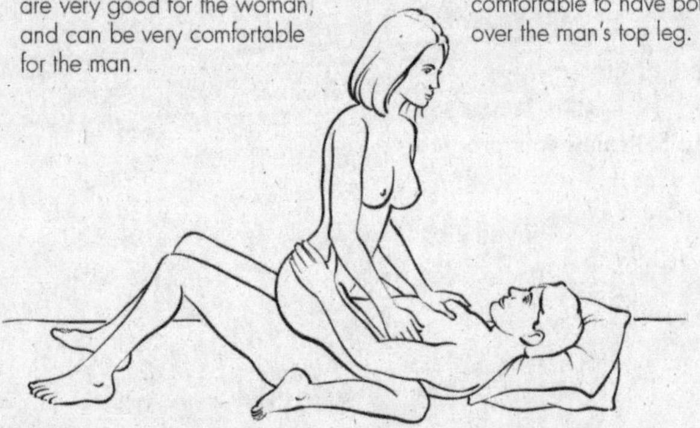

It is often best for the person in pain to let their partner take the dominant position on top and do the moving.

9. Guide to safe medicine use

This resource is to help you keep yourself **safe** and to help you **arrange a regular review by a prescribing healthcare professional**.

Safe medicine use

Ask about your medicines if you are prescribed them or buy them from a pharmacy.

- What does this medication do?
- How long will I need to use it?
- How and when should I take it?
- Should I avoid other medicines, drinks, foods or activities when I am taking this medicine?
- What are the possible risks or side-effects and what should I do if they happen to me?

And when you see your prescribing healthcare professional for a review:

- Share any questions or concerns about the medicines you are prescribed or buying – and ask about other options.
- Tell a healthcare professional about the medicines you are taking.
- Tell them if you think the medicines you are taking are not working or are giving you side-effects.
- Are you unsure how to take your medicines, or for how long? If so, ask.
- Ask if you need help getting a regular supply and regular review of your medicines.

10. Setback plan

In my setback plan I will try (use the above headings):

1. ______________________________

____

____

2. ______________________________

____

____

3. ______________________________

____

____

Now you have a setback plan how **confident** are you that you **can manage the next** setback?

0 1 2 3 4 5 6 7 8 9 10

Not at all confident — Extremely confident

If your confidence is low (less than 5), then review your plan →: page 319, and use the question 'What would my best friend suggest to improve my setback plan?'

11. Pleasurable activity list

Talk to friend on phone	Go to favourite café for coffee or tea
Go out and visit a friend	Go to a sporting event
Invite a friend to your house	Play a game with a friend
Send text message to a friend	Play Solitaire (with real cards)
Send e-mail or post to a friend	Go online to chat
Exercise	Look for blogs you like
Stretch your muscles	Visit your favourite websites
Go for a walk in a park or somewhere peaceful	Listen to a podcast (start downloading favourite podcasts)
Do yoga, tai chi, Pilates or take classes to learn	Sell something you don't want on the internet
Ride your bike	Create your own website or blog
Go for a jog	Join an internet dating service
Go for a swim	Buy something on the internet
Go for a hike	Do a puzzle with lots of pieces
Get a massage	Do a puzzle or sudoku
Go to a spa	Go get a pedicure or manicure

Get out of house, even if you just sit outside	Go to a magazine stand and peruse magazines
Go for a drive in your car, or on public transportation	Go to café or square and watch other people, imagine what they are thinking
Plan a trip to a place you've never been before	Go to library and check out books on topics, hobbies, places you are curious about
Make a cup of tea	Go to a bookstore and read
Cook your favourite meal	Go shopping
Cook a recipe you've never tried before	Go to a craft store and look around for ideas
Take a cooking class	Get a hair cut
Go out for something to eat	Learn a new language
Eat something you really like	Listen to a show in another language
Go outside and play with your pet	Sing or learn to sing
Borrow a friend's dog and take it to the park	Listen to upbeat, happy music (make list of songs, or a playlist)
Go outside and watch the birds or other animals	Turn on some loud music and dance around
Go to zoo or aquarium	Memorise lines from your favourite movie, play, song or poem
Watch a funny movie (start collecting funny movies)	Make a movie with your camera or video camera
Go to library or film place to rent a film	Make a list of celebrities you'd like to be friends with and say why

Go to cinema and watch whatever is playing	Join a public speaking group and write a speech
Listen to the radio	Participate in a local theatre group
Watch a specific show on television	Sing in a local choir
Paint a picture with a brush or fingers	Join a club
Knit, crochet, or sew – or learn how to	Plant a garden
Draw a picture	Plant plants for balcony or inside
Take photographs	Take a walk and look at other's gardens
Volunteer at a local organisation	Paint your nails
Visit a museum or local art gallery	Change your hair colour
Go to church, synagogue, temple or other place of worship	Work on your car, bicycle or motorcycle
Pray or meditate	Take a bubble bath or shower
Cut out pictures from old magazines and make a collage	Rub your feet and hands with lotion
Adapt a song with your own lyrics	Masturbate
Make a list of people you admire and want to be like	Have sex with someone you care about
Describe what you admire about these people	Sign up for class at a local school, college or online
Imagine how someone you admire would act/do in your life	Read your favourite book, magazine, newspaper, or poem

Make a list of places you'd like to visit nearby	Read a trashy magazine
Write a poem, story, play about your life or someone else's life	Write a letter or card to a friend or family member
Make a list of ten things you'd like to do before you die	Write things you like about yourself
Write a letter to someone who has made your life better and tell them why (you do not need to send it)	Write in your journal or diary about what happened today
Write about the craziest, funniest, or sexiest thing that has ever happened to you	Write a loving letter to yourself when you are feeling good and keep it to read when you are upset
Write a song	Make a list of ten things you are good at and keep it to read when you are upset
Play an instrument or learn how to play one	Start a collage of cartoons that make you laugh
Start a quote list, of quotes that inspire you and/or make you laugh	Create your own list of pleasurable activities
Organise a party	Other ideas:

Index

acceptance 4, 31–51, 317, 341
  case study 32–4, 39–40
  cycle of pain and non-acceptance 36, 37, 43
  defining 36
  exploring 35–7
  mindfulness for 36, 42–9
  of negative events 36
  ongoing journey of change 36, 38
  and openings for growth 38–41
  of reality 37
  skills of 37–8
  value of 31–5
activity *see* physical activity
acute pain 53, 62, 65–6
  acute pain puzzle 63–4
  characteristics of 62
  function of 62, 65, 66
  rest and 53
  time-limited 62
addiction problems 104–5, 294
adrenaline 49, 79, 241, 251, 264, 269, 276–7, 281, 342
aggression
  aggressive communication 218, 219
  feelings of 12
alcohol 269, 293, 294
'all or nothing' thinking 144
amitriptyline 205
anaesthetics 95
anger, frustration and irritability xix, 4, 12, 13, 15, 39, 99, 104, 267–89
  adrenaline rush 276–7, 281
  Anger Coping Plan 284–7, 288
  anticipating situations 281
  arousal 276–7
  case study 270–1, 281, 284–7
  checking for balanced thinking 285
  communicating feelings 282, 284–5
  exploring the effects 270–5
  and low mood 291
  management 276–89
  muscle tension and 273
  Out-Breath First skill 277, 281, 285
  physical symptoms 269, 270, 273
  seeing another point of view 282
  self-calming 277, 281, 285
  self-talk 278, 279, 280–1, 282
  time outs, taking 279, 281
  triggers 268–9
anti-depressants 205, 313–14

anxiety, worry and fears 4, 13, 99, 101, 103, 104, 177, 237–66
about life situation 238
about other people's perceptions of you 238
about pain itself 238
about physical symptoms 238
beneficial anxiety 240, 251
caffeine intake, limiting 264
case studies 243, 244, 247, 248–9, 252–4, 261–3
common worries and fears 238–9
coping self-talk 250–1, 266
fear of disability or being a burden 7
'fight or flight' survival response 276–7
Four-Steps-to-Balanced-Thinking 242–58, 266, 309, 369–72
letting go of fear 38
levels of 240
management 242–66
negative cycle of fear 242, 243
physical effects 238, 240, 241, 244, 251, 263
relaxation and unwinding 263, 266
safety behaviours 241–2
SMART goal-setting 260–3
unhelpful thinking and beliefs 241, 242, 245–9
'worry half-hour' 204
'worry'/'things to remember' notebook 202, 203
see also negative thinking patterns
apps 358–60
aromatherapy 179, 201, 337
art therapists 90
assertive communication 218, 219–24
'attacking' language, avoidance of 220
'broken record' skill 223
case study 222–3
expressing personal needs or concerns 219–20
with health professionals 220, 221
saying 'No' 220, 222–3
audio resources 357
Automatic Thought Tracker 243–5, 255, 266, 270, 274, 275, 276, 277, 280, 369
avoidance behaviours 258, 259

balance, problems with 21
balanced thinking 144, 249–54, 257–8, 314
'best friend questions' 250, 285, 311, 333
checking for 285
cycle of balanced thinking and balanced activity 259–60
see also Four-Steps-to-Balanced-Thinking
bath, taking a 201, 261–3, 337
bias against oneself 246
'bird therapy' 346
bites and stings 71
black-and-white thinking 247, 282, 285
bladder control, loss of 98
bowel control, loss of 98
brain
emotional areas 69, 70
focus of attention area 70
genetic programming 70–1
misinterpretation of pain 69, 71–2, 73, 74
natural opioids 49, 78, 342
neuroplasticity 74–5, 76
pain, experience of 55, 64, 66, 67, 68, 69–72, 73

pain memory areas 68, 70
'retraining the brain' 74–5, 76, 78, 79, 176, 177, 187
spatial area 70
thalamus (interpretation centre) 70
breathing
for anxiety management 263
diaphragm/belly breathing 178, 179
mindful breathing exercise 46, 48
Out-Breath First skill 277, 281, 285
relaxed 43, 178, 179, 182–3, 263, 336
unhelpful breathing patterns 177–8
Buddhism 42
burns 68

caffeine intake, limiting 201, 264
cannabis 293, 294
case histories
Jim xv–xvii, 3, 77–8, 97, 128, 129–30, 133, 143–4, 178, 180–1, 183, 195, 196–7, 208, 213–14, 224–5, 232, 233–4, 236, 243, 244, 247, 248–9, 252–4, 321, 323, 337
Maria 3, 8–9, 12–26, 58–9, 75, 270–1, 281, 284–7
Mo xviii–xx, 3, 32–4, 39–40, 48–9, 73, 79, 83, 93–4, 103, 112–16, 129, 131, 152–3, 158–60, 324, 325, 326–7, 329, 330, 331, 333, 335
Razia xiii–xv, 3, 56, 119–20, 141–2, 151–2, 171, 178, 184, 222–3, 261–3, 295–6, 299–305, 313–14, 321, 325–6, 337
catastrophising 246, 333
central nervous system 63
changing the impact of pain 6–30, 322
case study 8–9, 12–26
concerns about making changes 24–5
confidence level, rating 25, 26
hopeful about possibility of change 38
identifying targets for change 15–18, 20
importance of making changes, rating 25
readiness for change, rating 26
small changes 21
understanding the impact of pain 9–15
chemical injuries 68
chronic pain
acceptance of 31–51
brain chemistry 55, 64, 66, 67, 68, 69–72, 73
changing how you think about pain 74–5
characteristics 63
classified as a disease 54
control over your life, rating 6, 91
cure, letting go idea of 38, 54
effects on your life, assessing 9–15
holistic approach to pain management ix–x, 54
number of people affected by 57
puzzle of 2, 64
research into ix, 2
self-management, rewards of 7–8
cocaine 293
cognitive behavioural therapy (CBT) 85, 92, 100, 101, 103–4
see also Five-Areas tool

communication 4, 212–30
active listening 217
aggressive mode 218, 219
anger and frustration, communicating helpfully 282, 284–5
assertive 218, 219–24
case studies 213–14, 222–3, 224–5
with family and friends 213–14, 222–3, 225–7
having conversations 216–18, 224–5
with healthcare professionals 220, 221, 377
intimacy and 232–4
'listen slot', timed 217–18
passive mode 218, 219
problem areas 215–16, 225–6
professional support with 215
respectful 217, 218
rewards 227, 228, 230
skills 214–15
support for self-management through 227–9
talking about living with pain 229–30
tips 226–7
community mental health nurses 20
conclusions, jumping to 247, 285
confidence level rating 25, 26, 91, 106, 254
constipation 13, 113, 269
counsellors 90
craft activities 180–1
cure, letting go idea of 38, 54

daily activities
pacing *see* pacing
as part of setback plan 337
physical fitness, value of 154
relaxation sessions as part of 181, 184–5
depression *see* low mood and depression
describing your pain 57–61
in behaviour 60
in the body 60
case study 58–9
in life situation 60
in the mind 60
in moods 60
using Five-Areas tool 59–61
diary keeping 4
pacing diary 132–6
Physical Activity Diary 156–64, 206, 364–5
Positive Diary Log 283, 324–7, 325–6, 336
sleep diary 195–9, 367–8
disc, bulging 9
drug abuse 293, 294
dry mouth 113

eating disorders 99
Edison, Thomas 330–1
emotional distress 32, 99
see also grief and loss, feelings of; low mood and depression
endorphins 78
energy, boosting 127
energy, lack of 21, 269
see also tiredness
enjoyable activities
as part of setback plan 336, 337
sociable activities 111, 127, 167, 345–6
suggestions for 379–82
to combat low mood 298–9, 314
exercise
exercise classes 168
stretching exercises 19, 62, 75, 76, 78, 79, 333, 336
see also physical activity

expectations and reality, gap between 32, 33, 34
see also acceptance
extreme statements and rules 247

falls, reducing chance of 168
family
communication with 213–14, 222–3, 225–7
health professionals' support for 100
see also relationships
fears *see* anxiety, worry and fears
fibromyalgia xiv, 295
'fight or flight' survival response 276–7
fitness *see* physical activity
fitness instructors 90
Five Areas tool 54, 98, 99, 101, 111, 340, 363
benefits of relaxation 188
describing pain using 59–61
exploring impact of pain 9–15
exploring low mood/depression 294–7
identifying targets for change 15–18
flexibility 19, 129, 170, 259
stretching exercises 19, 62, 75, 76, 78, 79, 333, 336
fortune telling 246
Four-Steps-to-Balanced-Thinking 242–58, 266, 309, 369–72
Automatic Thought Tracker 243–5, 255, 266, 270, 274, 275, 276, 277, 280, 369
balanced thinking questions 250
case study 247, 248–9, 252–4
challenging negative thoughts 248–9, 256–7, 309, 314
for low mood and depression 309–12
negative thinking styles, exploring 245–7, 256
practising balanced thinking 249–54, 257–8, 311, 314
frustration *see* anger, frustration and irritability
future, looking to the 319–47
life journey, guiding 340–6
long-term goals 324
Positive Diary Log 324–7
problem-solving skills 204, 327–31, 375
ten keys to happier living 346
tips 339
see also setback plans

gabapentin 205, 269
general practitioners (GPs) 20, 85, 86, 87
role 87, 90–1
skills and pain management 87
support for self-management 87
genetic data 70–1
goals 110–24
breaking down into smaller steps 118–20
building on goals 123
case studies 112–16, 119–20
goal ladder 118–19, 120, 122, 261, 366
goal-setting 110, 111, 112–23, 124, 146, 235
helpfulness in pain management 110–11
'overachieving' pattern, setbacks and 121
physical activity goals 155, 324
revising and adjusting 117
rewards 110, 111, 112, 123, 124, 142, 169, 227, 228, 230, 283, 289, 299, 331

self-check on progress 123
setbacks, dealing with 123
sharing with other people 117
short and long-term 111–12, 324
SMART goals 115–19, 155, 180, 260–3, 324, 366
grief and loss, feelings of 4, 36, 39, 100, 104, 290, 316
normality of 292
see also low mood and depression
group treatment
pain management programmes (PMPs) 105–8
self-help groups 90, 106, 355–6
guilt, feelings of 293, 296, 303

hamstrings, tight 79
health coaches 90, 170
healthcare professionals 4, 20, 82–109
cognitive behavioural therapists 85
communication with 220, 221, 377
general practitioners (GPs) 20, 85, 86, 87, 90–1
nurse practitioners 85, 87
occupational therapists 20
pain management programmes (PMPs) 105–8
pain medicine specialists 85, 88, 95–8, 100
pain specialist nurses 85, 89, 94–5
pharmacists 85
physiotherapists xv, xvii, 20, 83, 85, 88, 91–4, 97, 100, 170
primary care nurses/nurse practitioners 20, 90–1
psychologists 85, 98–100, 101, 215
skills and pain management 87–9
standards and quality of care 82, 86
support for self-management 87–9
talking therapists 85, 340
working with 82, 83, 84
heroin 293, 294
holistic approach to chronic pain management ix–x, *see also* Five Areas tool

independence, loss of 100
inflammation 67
injections 96, 97
'inner healing' 38
International Association for the Study of Pain (ISAP) 52, 54
International Classification of Disease 54
irritability *see* anger, frustration and irritability
isolation and loneliness 214

life situation 9, 14, 60
life journey, guiding 340–6
past life events, exploration of 104
problem-solving skills 204, 327–31, 375
ten keys to happier living 346
traumatic life experiences 99
worries about 238
see also acceptance; anger, frustration and irritability; anxiety, worry and fears; grief and loss, feelings of; low mood and depression; relationships
loss of feeling in arms or legs 98

loving-kindness towards oneself and others 341–2
guided meditation script 342–5
see also self-compassion
low mood and depression xv, xix, 4, 13, 19, 90, 98, 99, 104, 207, 290–318
Activity Plan 300–9, 314, 373–4
case study 295–6, 299–305, 313–14
challenging automatic unhelpful thinking 309, 314
effects of 292–3
excessive low mood 292
factors affecting 290–1
help and support 294, 315–16
low mood cycle 291
management 298–312
medication 313–14
negative mental filter 309
normality of low mood 292
oversleeping and 207
pain, impact of 290–1
planning enjoyable activities 298–9, 314
suicidal thoughts 315–16
symptoms 292, 293
using Five-Areas tool to understand 294–7
see also grief and loss, feelings of; negative thinking patterns

medication
addiction problems 104–5
anti-depressants 205, 313–14
injections 96, 97
insufficient pain relief 21
long-term use of 3
night-time 202
reducing 126, 313
review 313–14, 377
safe medicine use 377
side effects 3, 21, 85, 96, 113, 191–2, 205, 269, 291, 293, 294
trial periods 96, 104
see also opioids
meditation script 342–5
mental health symptoms 99, 100
CBT for 99, 104
see also anger, frustration and irritability; anxiety and worry; low mood and depression; panic attacks; post-traumatic stress disorder
mind reading 246
mindfulness 4, 179, 341
for acceptance 36, 42–9
and adrenaline reduction 49
for anxiety management 263, 266
apps 48
balancing 'reasonable' and 'emotional' thinking 43
being in the present moment 44–5
benefits of 42
breathing exercise 46, 48
case study 48–9
daily practice 49
exercises 46–7
mindful movement 48
and natural opioid release 49
non-judgmental 44, 48
non-judgmental exercise 47
observation exercise 46–7
observing 44, 48
skills 44–5
'wise mind' thinking approach 43
money worries 22, 238, 269
moods 9, 13, 21, 60
brighter 19, 126

factors affecting 269
management 151, 154, 216
mood change 243, 310
physical activity, benefits of 151
poor sleep and 192
see also anger, frustration and irritability; anxiety, worry and fears; low mood and depression
morphine 105, 293
muscle strengthening activities 155, 170, 259
muscle tension 174, 176–7
anger, effect of 273
body scanning 182
letting go 182, 281
music 167, 179, 202, 336

nature, connecting with 179, 346
negative thinking patterns 13, 43
anxiety and 241, 242, 245–9
automatic 256, 309
bias against oneself 246
black-and-white thinking 247, 282, 285
catastrophising 246, 333
challenging 248–9, 256–7, 309, 310–11, 314
conclusions, jumping to 247, 285
distortions 245
exploring 245–7, 310
extreme statements and rules 247
fortune telling 246
getting stuck in 39
low moods and 291
mind reading 246
mindfulness for 45
negative mental filter 246, 303, 309
personalisation 247
and physical tension 43
'reasonable' 245, 309
repetitive 245, 309
responsibility, unfair 247
sexual relationships and 236
using the Positive Diary Log to challenge 326–7
see also Four-Steps-to-Balanced-Thinking
nerve fibre sensors 65, 66–8, 76
change in sensitivity 66–7
damage, and resultant pain 68
over-sensitivity 67–8
pain 'memory', replaying 68
problems with 67–8
nerve networks 63, 64, 66, 74–5, 79
neuralgia 68
neuropathic pain 68, 105
neuroplasticity 74–5, 76
nortriptyline 205
numbness 98
nurse practitioners 85
role 87
skills and pain management 87
support for self-management 87

Obsessive Compulsive Disorder 99
occupational therapists 20
opioids
abuse of 293
addiction to 105
deaths as a result of (US) ix
drowsiness 205
effect on mood 269, 293, 294
endorphins 78
long-term use of 3
natural 49, 78, 342
osteoporosis 9
Out-Breath First skill 277, 281, 285
oxycodone 293

pacing 39, 62, 125–49, 335
active self-management skill 125–6
balanced thinking requirement 144
benefits of 126–7
case studies 77–8, 128, 129–32, 133, 141–2, 143–4, 321
Daily Pacing Plan 138–44
goal-setting 146
involving others 143–4, 146
matching activity to effort levels 137–8, 145, 146
mixed pacing style ('boom and bust') 77, 129, 131, 302
'must'/'should', replacing with 'could' 144, 145
overactive pacing 128, 130–1, 143, 145
prioritising activities 145
rest periods 145
rewards 142
self-check on progress 145–6
sexual relationships 234–5
timing activities 145
tracking activities 132–6
underactive pacing 129
pain
brain chemistry 55, 64, 65, 66, 67, 68, 69–72, 73
changed understandings of 53
changing the impact of 6–30
defining 52–3
describing to someone else 57–61
knowing more about 52–81
nerve fibre sensitivity and 65, 66–8, 76
pain cycle 27
shifting main focus of attention away from 62, 63
see also acute pain; chronic pain
pain management programmes (PMPs) 105–8
case study 107
community programmes 106
functions 106–7
outcomes 108
pain medicine specialists 85, 95–8, 100
case study 97
investigation of symptoms 98
medicine trials 96, 97
person-centred assessment 96
role 88, 95–6
skills and pain management 88
support for self-management 88
pain specialist nurses 85
role 89, 94–5
skills and pain management 89, 95
support for self-management 89, 95
panic attacks 99, 104
past life events, exploration of 104
personal trainers 170
personalisation 247
pessimism 292
see also low mood and depression
phantom limb pain 64, 68
pharmacists 20, 85
physical activity 4, 150–73
apps 358–60
avoidance 259
on bad pain days 151
balancing activity and rest 170
barriers to becoming more physically active 164–6, 227–8
benefits of 154, 156
case studies 151–3, 158–60, 171
cycle of balanced thinking and balanced activity 259–60
daily 154

enjoyable activities 111, 127, 167, 298–9, 314, 336, 337, 345–6, 379–82
exercise classes 168
exercise videos and apps 168
fitting into daily/weekly life 167–8, 170
GP, consulting 155
gradual increase in 168, 170
key steps to making changes 167–8
mindful movement 48
moderate intensity activity 154, 155, 157
muscle or joint aches 170
for muscle strength 155
outdoor gyms 155
as part of setback plan 337
Physical Activity Diary 156–64, 206, 364–5
rewards 169, 228
self-check on progress 169
SMART goals 155, 324
sociable activities 111, 127, 167, 345–6
structured programmes 170
value of in managing chronic pain 150–1
vigorous intensity activity 155
weekly target 154–5
see also pacing
physiotherapists xv, xvii, 20, 83, 85, 100, 170
case studies 93–4, 97
preparing for your assessment 94
role 88, 91–4
skills and pain management 88, 91–2
support for self-management 88, 92
Pilates 168, 179
Positive Diary Log 283, 324–7, 336
case studies 325–6
post-traumatic stress disorder 104, 186
pregabalin 269
primary care nurses/nurse practitioners 20, 90–1
see also pain specialist nurses
prioritising activities 145, 333
problem-solving skills 204, 327–31, 375
acceptance that a problem is not always changeable 327
case study 329, 330, 331
choosing a solution and acting on it 330
exploring advantages and disadvantages of solutions 329
listing possible solutions 329
recognising and defining the problem 328–9
reviewing progress 330–1
psychiatrists 100
role 104–5
psychologists 85, 215
reasons for working with 101
referral to 100
role 98–100

rehabilitation specialists *see* physiotherapists
relationships
difficulties xix–xx, 21, 269, 273
impact of low moods on 293
sexual relations and intimacy xvii, 231–6
worries over others' perceptions 238
see also communication
relaxation 4, 78, 174–89
for anxiety management 263, 266

apps and downloads 181, 185
barriers to 183–4
before bedtime 201–2
body scanning 182
breathing, relaxed 43, 178, 179, 182–3, 263, 336
case studies 178, 180–1, 183, 184
drowsiness and 186
exploring possibilities for 179, 180–1, 186
Five Areas tool 188
mental and physical sensations 175
muscle relaxation 182, 281
odd or distressing thoughts or images 185–6
as part of daily routine 184–5
as part of setback plan 337
professional advice 186
quick relaxation 182
reminders 183
'retraining the brain' 176, 177, 187
self-check on progress 187
sessions 185–6
SMART goals 180
'time-out' relaxation 181–2
value of in pain management 174–5, 176–7

resources 5, 349–56

rest
helpful for acute pain 53
rest periods during daily activities 145, 170
unhelpful for chronic pain 53, 73
see also relaxation; sleep

rewards 110, 112, 123, 124, 142, 169, 227, 228, 230, 283, 289, 299, 339
creative 331
helpfulness in pain management 111

safety behaviours 241–2, 258, 259

scar tissue 73, 76

self-care cycle 27–8, 93, 322–3

self-care skills *see* goals; pacing; physical activity; self-talk; sleep

self-compassion 49, 78, 100, 299, 336, 341–2, 353

self-help books 357–8

self-help groups 90, 106
websites 355–6

self-hypnosis 179

self-talk
for anger management 278, 279, 280–1, 282
case study 79
positive 79, 250–1, 266, 336

setback plans 252, 285, 320, 331–8, 378
case studies 253, 333, 335, 337
enjoyable activities 337
ideas 336–7
key areas, focus on 332–3
physical activities 337
relaxation 337
reviewing and adjusting 339
sharing with others 334
usefulness of 332

setbacks 4, 121, 123, 151, 177, 249, 332
see also setback plans

sexual relations and intimacy xvii, 231–6
case study 232, 233–4, 236
communication, sensitive 232–4
goal-setting 235
impact of low moods on 293
pacing 234–5
pain-free 235
practice 235
problems 21, 213–14, 231–2

sexual activity, avoidance of 213–14, 232
sexual positions 376
unhelpful thoughts and feelings 236
value of in pain management 232
shingles 68
sleep 190–211
amount of sleep required 193–4, 200
assessing current sleep pattern 194–5
bedrooms 181, 202, 203
bedtime routine, establishing 199, 200, 201–2
case studies 195, 196–7, 208
daytime naps 197, 200–1
good sleep, effects of 193
improving sleep patterns 4, 126, 199–208, 210
medication side effects and 191–2, 202, 205
mobile devices, switching off 202, 207
mood, effect of poor sleep on 192
poor sleep patterns xiv–xv, xvi–xvii, xx, 13, 21, 72, 101, 104, 112–13
problems with sleep 190–2
self-check on progress 209
sleep diary 195–9, 367–8
too much sleep 205–7
value of good sleep in pain management 190–3
wakefulness, dealing with 203–4, 333
winding-down routine 201–2
worries and unhelpful thoughts, dealing with 204–5
sleep apnoea 206
SMART goals 115–19, 155, 180, 260–3, 324, 366
smoking 293
sociable activities 111, 127, 167, 345–6
social workers 90
spiritual or religious beliefs 38
spondylosis 9
stair climbing 93, 103
stiffness 13, 19, 75, 151, 259
stretching exercises 19, 62, 75, 76, 78, 79, 333, 336
suicidal thoughts 315–16
support *see* healthcare professionals; relationships; self-help groups
swimming 111

t'ai chi 76, 168, 179
talking therapists 85, 101–4, 215, 340
assessment session 101–2
case study 103
cognitive behavioural therapy (CBT) 85, 92, 98, 100, 101, 103–4
reasons for working with 101
role 89, 98–100
skills and pain management 89
support for self-management 89
thalamus 70
thinking patterns 4, 60
'all or nothing' thinking 144
Automatic Thought Tracker 243–4, 255, 266, 270, 274, 275, 276, 277, 369
balanced thinking 144, 249–54, 257–8, 311
'must'/'should', replacing with 'could' 144, 145
negative *see* negative thinking patterns
see also moods

tiredness 21, 72, 104, 126, 177, 269, 290, 292
see also relaxation; sleep
traumatic life experiences 99

visualisation 177

walking 62, 335
difficulties in 21, 98
pacing 79, 335

websites 349–56, 358–60
'What are my Health Needs now?' 20, 21–2
work, loss of 14, 22, 100, 238
World Health Organisation 54
worry *see* anxiety, worry and fears

yoga 76, 168, 179

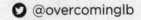